LIFT YOUR MOOD WITH
POWER
FOODS

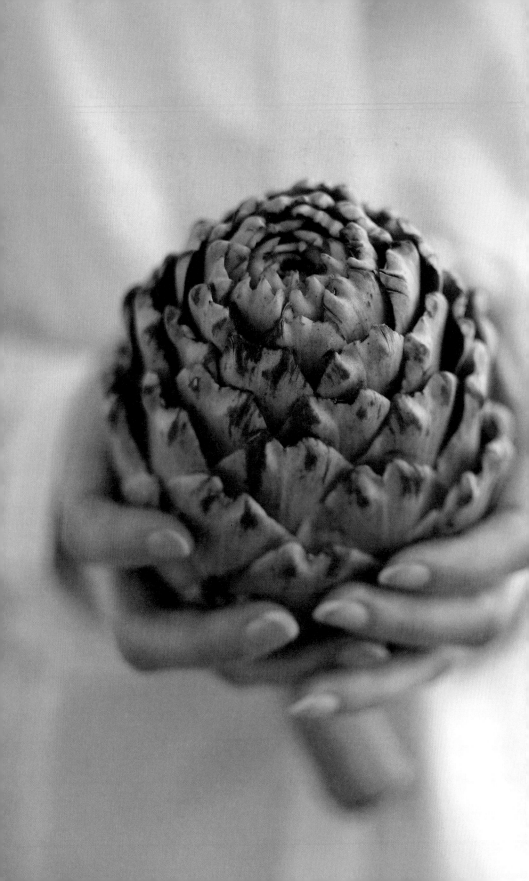

LIFT YOUR MOOD WITH

POWER

FOODS

MORE T   IPES
TO CHAI

NUTRITIONAL CONSULTANT

CHRISTINE
BAILEY

DUNCAN BAIRD PUBLISHERS

LONDON

LIFT YOUR MOOD WITH POWER FOODS

First published in the United Kingdom
and Ireland in 2014 by
Duncan Baird Publishers, an imprint of
Watkins Publishing Limited
Sixth Floor, 75 Wells Street
London W1T 3QH

A member of Osprey Group

Managing Editor: Sarah Epton
Editors: James Hodgson and Krissy Mallett
Designer: Clare Thorpe
Commissioned Photography: William Lingwood
Photography Assistant: Emma Bentham-Wood
Stylists: David Morgan and Helen Trent

A CIP record for this book is available from the
British Library

ISBN: 978-1-84899-080-7

10 9 8 7 6 5 4 3 2 1

Typeset in Warnock Pro and Omnes
Colour reproduction by PDQ, UK
Printed in China

PUBLISHER'S NOTE

The information in this book is not intended as
a substitute for professional medical advice and
treatment. If you are pregnant or breastfeeding or
have any special dietary requirements or medical
conditions, it is recommended that you consult
a medical professional before following any of
the information or recipes contained in this
book. Watkins Publishing Limited, or any other
persons who have been involved in working on
this publication, cannot accept responsibility for
any errors or omissions, inadvertent or not, that
may be found in the recipes or text, nor for any
problems that may arise as a result of preparing
one of these recipes or following the advice
contained in this work.

NOTES ABOUT THE RECIPES

Unless otherwise stated:
Use medium fruit and vegetables
Use medium organic or free-range eggs
Use fresh ingredients, including herbs and chillies
Use coconut oil for cooking (olive oil can be used
    if coconut oil is not available)
Do not mix metric and imperial measurements
1 tsp = 5ml   1 tbsp = 15ml   1 cup = 250ml

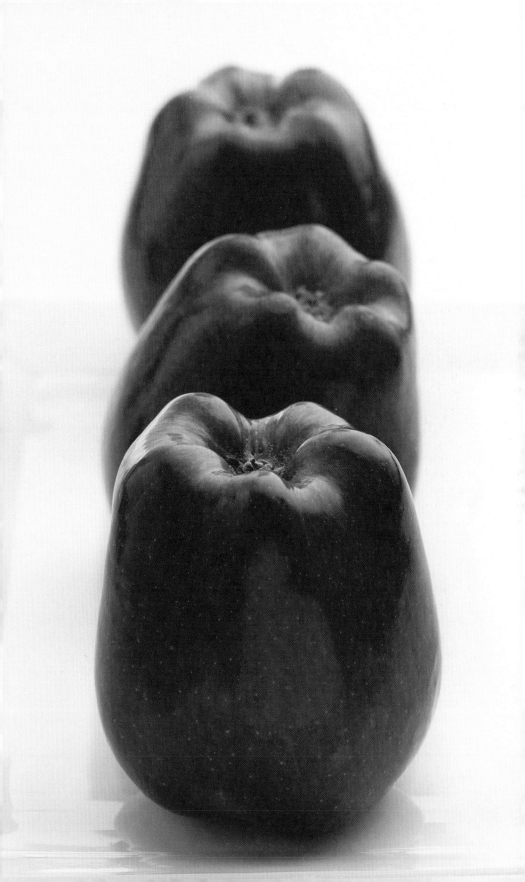

CONTENTS

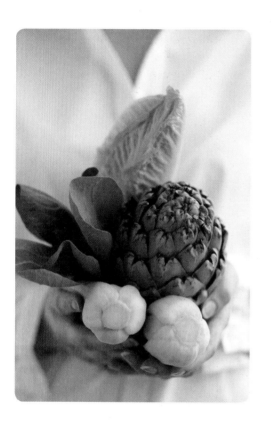

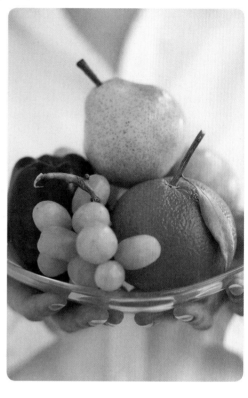

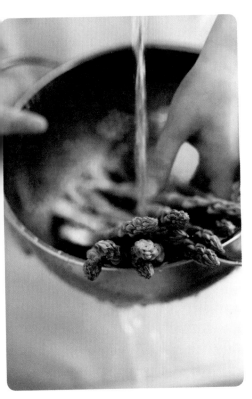
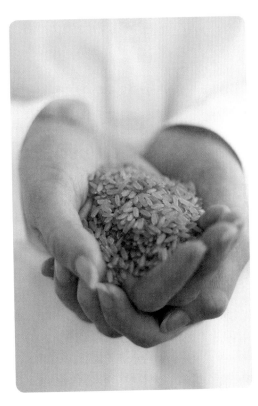

INTRODUCTION

We all want to feel happy, alert, motivated and full of vitality. Yet in reality many of us find ourselves struggling with low mood, depression, anxiety, lack of energy, and poor focus and concentration on a daily basis. In addition, with an increasing number of people being diagnosed with dementia and Alzheimer's, many are concerned about mental decline – from misplacing items and bouts of occasional forgetfulness to lapses in concentration and loss of mental agility.

Yet it is possible to feel positive and promote optimal brain health even as we age. And we can achieve this not through "pick-me-ups" such as caffeine or alcohol, but through a lifestyle and diet that supports an optimal balance of key brain messengers. The information in this book will show you how to keep these messengers (known as neurotransmitters, or NTs) in the right balance through food and nutrition. It will enable you to promote optimal brain health, reduce the risk of mental decline and keep you sharp and alert. While genes may play their part, we all have the capacity to alter our current state of well-being – both physical and mental – through dietary and lifestyle changes. Some of these, such as cutting out caffeine, alcohol or sugary snacks, may feel tough at first – we often use these treats as milestones in our busy days, but if you are looking to improve your health you will need to make some changes. Collapsing on the sofa with a glass of wine after coming home from work and/or getting the children to bed can be a hard habit to break. However, when temptation strikes, remind yourself that the sooner you start implementing healthy changes the sooner you will experience positive thinking, improved mood and increased energy.

This book is aimed at anyone who finds themselves constantly tired, unmotivated, low in mood, anxious, stressed, or suffering from poor sleep or reduced cognitive function. Chapter 1, "The Physiology of Melancholy", includes information to help you ascertain whether there are underlying nutritional imbalances that may be affecting your mood and energy levels and offers strategies for addressing those imbalances. Chapter 2, "Mood's Many Guises", gives practical nutritional solutions designed to alleviate various mood-related conditions.

In Chapter 3, "Feel-Good Food", you'll find clear guidelines on key foods to include in your diet as well as a wide selection of simple, quick and healthy recipes to use every day. All the recipes feature ingredients that are widely available in supermarkets or health-food stores and they provide a range of nutritional benefits. Remember, however, that optimal brain health relies on lifestyle changes as well as dietary approaches, and exercise, rest and recovery are discussed in the final chapter, "The Whole Picture".

OUR BRAIN MESSENGERS: NEUROTRANSMITTERS

How we think, feel and behave on a daily basis is intimately influenced by the balance of various chemical messengers (the neurotransmitters) in our brain. When this process is working optimally, our brain chemistry is said to be balanced and we respond appropriately and positively to the world around us.

For optimal brain health we need the correct synthesis of these brain chemicals as well as their effective transmission along neurons. Neurons are tiny nerve cells in the brain that send and receive messages. They are also mood control centres that influence our feelings as well as behaviours. Neurons connect to each other via thread-like branches known as dendrites. Our chemical messengers, the neurotransmitters, travel along these neurons and are transmitted between one neuron to the next at gaps known as synapses.

For successful transmission a neuron produces the neurotransmitter, which is sent across a synapse and attaches to a receptor site on the receiving neuron. This in turn activates the receptor, allowing the chemical message to travel along the neuron until it reaches another synapse, creating the release of another neurotransmitter. So for optimal balanced brain health it is important that:

- the right level of neurotransmitters is maintained
- the neurotransmitters are able to travel effectively along neurons
- the neurotransmitters can travel between neurons, across synapses
- the neurotransmitters can attach to and activate the relevant receptors on the neurons' membranes
- the neurotransmitters are effectively removed when they have fulfilled their role

All of these actions require the correct amount of certain nutrients to be in place.

UNDERSTANDING OUR KEY NEUROTRANSMITTERS

While there are actually hundreds of different neurotransmitters there are some key ones found to influence how we think and feel:

Dopamine, adrenalin and *noradrenalin*: These are our feel-good neurotransmitters helping to keep us energized, motivated and stimulated.

Serotonin: Often described as the "happy" neurotransmitter. Serotonin is further metabolized to melatonin, an important antioxidant hormone that promotes sleep.

Gamma-aminobutyric acid (GABA): This quietens the brain, reducing anxiety and encouraging a sense of calm.

Acetylcholine: For memory, mental alertness and skeletal muscle function.

Endorphins: These work like opiate drugs, relieving pain and promoting euphoria.

Glutamate: Highly stimulatory and can lead to over-excitation.

Taurine: This helps promote GABA and thereby brings about calmness.

KEEPING IN BALANCE

Neurotransmitters are manufactured in the neurons from amino acids, which are the building blocks of protein. The following table lists the key amino acids each neuro-transmitter needs, as well as highlighting signs and symptoms of typical imbalances.

NEUROTRANSMITTER	AMINO ACID BUILDING BLOCK	SIGNS OF IMBALANCES
Adrenalin and Noradrenalin	Phenylalanine Tyrosine	LOW LEVELS Poor cognitive function Poor concentration HIGH LEVELS Palpitations Cardiovascular problems Panic attacks
Dopamine	Phenylalanine Tyrosine	LOW LEVELS Poor concentration Poor memory Boredom, apathy and low enthusiasm Depressed feelings Low drive and motivation Low libido or impotence Mental and physical fatigue Tendency to develop addictions HIGH LEVELS Psychosis Compulsive tendencies Anxiety Aggression Low pain threshold
GABA	Taurine Glutamine	LOW LEVELS Anxiety, nervousness Phobias

GABA (continued)		Feeling stressed, being overwhelmed Trouble relaxing Stiffness, shaking Sleep problems
Glutamate	Glutamate Glutamine	HIGH LEVELS Neuro-degenerative diseases Hyperactivity Migraines Poor concentration Irritability Aggression Mood swings
Serotonin	Tryptophan	LOW LEVELS Depression Insomnia/sleep problems Irritability/impatience Self-destructiveness Thinking about the same things over and over Low self-esteem/confidence Feeling worse in and disliking dark weather Chronic pain/PMS Eating disorders HIGH LEVELS Agitation Confusion Delirium Tachycardia (fast/irregular heartbeat) Blood-pressure changes Sweating
Acetylcholine	Choline, DMAE (Dimethylaminoethanol)	LOW LEVELS Poor concentration Poor memory Forgetting where you put things Slowed and/or confused thinking Difficulty finding the right words Increased risk of dementia

Too much or too little of one or more of these neurotransmitters will cause an imbalance in brain chemistry and potentially a range of signs or symptoms.

HOW NUTRITION CAN HELP

The production of neurotransmitters is not just dependent on providing the right building blocks (amino acids). It also depends on how efficient you are in converting the amino acids into neurotransmitters. This requires an array of vitamins and minerals that can aid a process known as methylation. Methylation is a series of chemical reactions that help create and balance neurotransmitters, build cells and protect your brain from damage (*see* box, page 34).

For effective transmission neurotransmitters need to bind to receptors situated within the membrane of the neuron. Essential fats and phospholipids are required to form these receptors as well as the protective myelin sheath around the neurons. Therefore it is important your diet is rich in the right healthy fats (*see* pages 38–43). The essential fats that make up the brain cell membranes and receptors are vulnerable to damage and oxidation. Protecting your brain health therefore requires a plentiful supply of antioxidants (*see* page 89–91). Key antioxidants include the following:

• vitamins A, C and E
• alpha lipoic acid, glutathione and N-acetyl cysteine (NAC)
• phytonutrients – found in plants (fruits, vegetables, herbs and spices)

The recipes and diet plans in this book have been designed to provide the full range of vitamins, minerals, essential fats and antioxidants you need to keep your neurotransmitters in balance. They are also intended to help your body to regulate physiological processes such as inflammation, blood-glucose production, detoxification and adrenal function that are vital in balancing brain chemistry – and therefore your mood. The significance of the gut–brain connection (*see* pages 56–7) and the role of nutrition in its operation cannot be overstated.

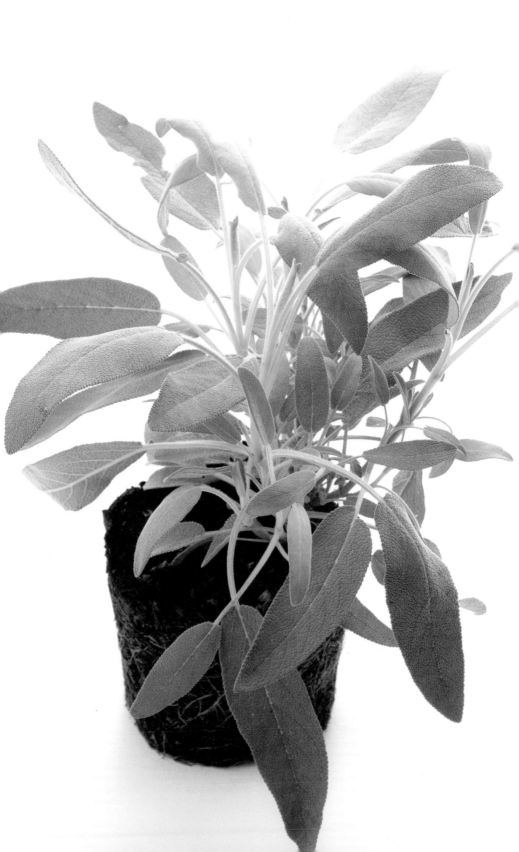

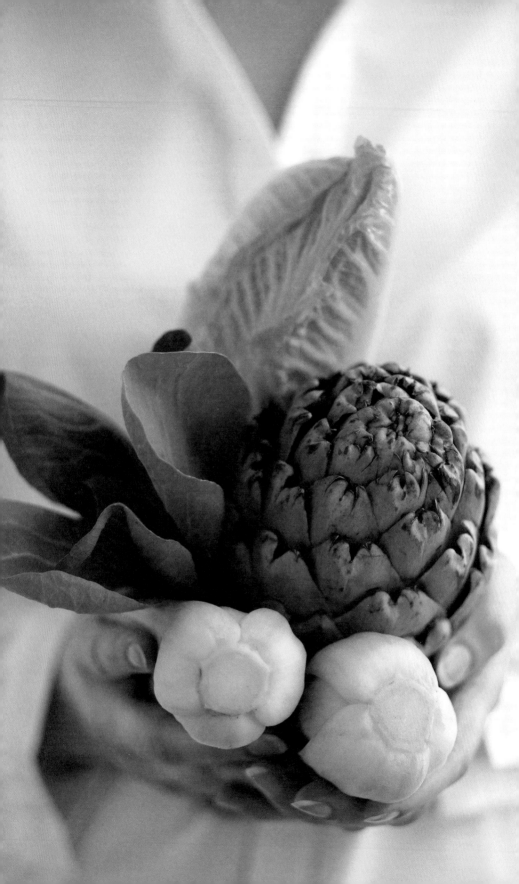

THE PHYSIOLOGY
OF MELANCHOLY

As many of the ancient sages knew, balance is crucial if you are to maintain good health. Understanding exactly how your body systems work is an important first step in redressing any hidden nutritional imbalances that may be undermining the myriad physical processes that govern your moods.

Feeling good in your body, mind and soul calls for balance across all aspects of your life, including your diet. In this chapter, we examine how important body systems – such as blood-sugar balance, stress response and detoxification – work, and explore why if any of your body's finely tuned mechanisms are even slightly off key, symptoms such as low mood, insomnia and cravings may result. We explore how your diet and lifestyle may be affecting your body functions – and therefore your moods and energy – and also discover ways of supporting the body systems that affect your mental health through a few simple dietary changes.

BLOOD-SUGAR BALANCE

Do you suffer from recurrent dips in mood, concentration and energy? Do you reach for a sugary snack or a cup of coffee to "pick you up", only to find you feel grumpy and exhausted again shortly afterwards? By improving your diet and eating patterns you can help balance your blood sugar, which in turn can improve your energy levels and mood.

On the list below, tick those symptoms or habits that apply to you on a regular basis:

- ☐ fatigue
- ☐ irritability/foggy head
- ☐ cravings for sweet foods, carbohydrates or sugary drinks
- ☐ cravings for caffeine and/or cigarettes
- ☐ need to snack regularly
- ☐ lapses in mood/concentration/memory
- ☐ difficulty making decisions
- ☐ light-headedness/fainting/feeling shaky without food
- ☐ sweating for no apparent reason
- ☐ difficulty getting to sleep, or waking in the night
- ☐ headaches
- ☐ palpitations
- ☐ regularly skipping breakfast or other meals
- ☐ mood swings
- ☐ difficulty getting going in the morning
- ☐ energy dips or slumps

If you ticked six or more of the above symptoms, you may need help in keeping your blood sugar balanced.

In order to maintain even blood-sugar levels, we need a full range of nutrients, which are best obtained from a varied, balanced diet.

BITE-SIZE SOLUTION

Breakfast's name comes from breaking your overnight fast – providing the brain and body with fuel to get the day started. Skipping breakfast can result in fluctuating blood-sugar levels and cravings. But ditch the sugary cereals and toast. Choose a protein-based breakfast to kick start your metabolism and keep you feeling satisfied through the morning.

NUTRIENTS FOR BLOOD-SUGAR BALANCE

The following nutrients are particularly important if you are looking to balance and maintain even blood-sugar levels:

NUTRIENT	RICH FOOD SOURCES
Protein	Dairy products, eggs, fish, meat, poultry, soya
Magnesium	Almonds, fish, green leafy vegetables, molasses, nuts, soya beans, sunflower seeds, wheatgerm
Chromium	Beef, brewer's yeast, chicken, eggs, fish, fruit, milk products, potatoes, whole grains
Vitamin B1	Beef kidney and liver, brewer's yeast, chickpeas, kidney beans, pork, rice bran, salmon, soya beans, sunflower seeds, wheatgerm, whole grain wheat and rye
Vitamin B2	Almonds, brewer's yeast, cheese, chicken, wheatgerm
Vitamin B3	Beef liver, brewer's yeast, chicken, fish, sunflower seeds, turkey
Vitamin B5	Blue cheese, brewer's yeast, corn, eggs, lentils, liver, lobster, meats, peanuts, peas, soya beans, sunflower seeds, wheatgerm, whole grains
Vitamin C	Blackcurrants, broccoli, Brussels sprouts, cabbage, grapefruit, green peppers, guava, kale, lemons, oranges, papaya, potatoes, spinach, strawberries, tomatoes, watercress
Vanadium	Buckwheat, fish, mushrooms, parsley, shellfish, soya
Manganese	Barley, buckwheat, dried fruit, green leafy vegetables, nuts, oats, seaweed, whole grains
Vitamin D	Herring, mackerel, porcini or shiitake mushrooms
Omega 3 fatty acids	Herring, mackerel, sardines, trout, wild salmon, chia seeds, flaxseed, pumpkin seeds, walnuts
Alpha lipoic acid	Leafy green vegetables, organic kidney, liver
Zinc	Lean cuts of beef, pork, lamb and venison, calf's liver, crab, poultry, sea vegetables, seeds, whole grains

If your diet is high in carbohydrates and refined sugary foods, this will raise glucose levels, which in turn triggers the release of insulin and sends out excess glucose from the blood to be stored as fat. Gradually the receptors for insulin become less sensitive to overuse and your body is required to produce more and more insulin, a disorder known as insulin resistance. The result can be devastating to brain health. Firstly as you become more and more insensitive to insulin your blood-sugar levels will remain raised and this can damage brain cells. High blood glucose also results in glycation – a process that also damages your brain cells and can in turn result in poor cognitive function and mental decline. As insulin resistance is associated with the biochemical imbalances of increased oxidation, inflammation and glycation, if you suspect you have problems balancing your blood-sugar levels you should take steps to resolve this as soon as possible.

In addition to the effects of glycation, as glucose is taken from the blood and dumped as fat not only do you put on weight but you will experience a dip in energy levels as blood glucose falls. This can leave you feeling tired, lacking in energy, irritable, grumpy and prone to mood swings. It will also result in cravings for something sweet, sugary or carbohydrate-rich. This in turn will result in fluctuations in blood-sugar levels through the day and subsequent effects on your mood and energy.

Maintaining an even blood-sugar level is, therefore, one of the most important factors in improving our moods.

BRAIN FUEL

Fluctuating blood-sugar levels also affect your concentration and mental performance. While the best fuel for the brain cells is glucose, for your brain to function optimally it requires a *steady* supply of glucose and nutrients. For this to happen it is important that glucose is derived from slow-releasing, complex carbohydrates.

Carbohydrate-rich foods are often classed as simple or complex. Simple carbohydrates are generally refined and broken down and absorbed more quickly than others. Complex carbohydrates include whole grains, vegetables, beans and pulses, which tend to be higher in naturally occurring fibre, and therefore provide the body with a more steady supply of glucose.

GLYCAEMIC INDEX (GI) AND GLYCAEMIC LOAD (GL)

An effective way to evaluate how quickly carbohydrates are broken down into glucose in the body is to measure their glycaemic index (GI) and glycaemic load (GL). GI and GL are important concepts to grasp if you need to balance your blood-sugar levels.

WHAT CARBOHYDRATES CAN I EAT FOR BLOOD-SUGAR BALANCE?

Base your meals around low-glycaemic foods, especially vegetables, and include plenty of lean protein with each meal. The following list highlights the best carbohydrates to include.

CARBOHYDRATES TO EAT IN ABUNDANCE
(Eat daily)

Low-glycaemic vegetables: asparagus, broccoli, kale, spinach, cabbage, Brussels sprouts and sea vegetables (nori, hijiki, arame and wakame).

CARBOHYDRATES TO EAT IN MODERATION
(Limit to a portion of whole grains or starchy vegetables daily; limit fruit to two portions)

Whole grains: whole-grain rice, black and red rice, quinoa, amaranth, buckwheat, rye, wheat and oats – one portion is 50–60g (1¾oz–2¼oz/⅓ cup) cooked.

Starchy vegetables: squash and pumpkin, potatoes, sweetcorn and root vegetables such as beetroot – one portion is 100–125g (3½–4½oz/½ cup) cooked.

Beans and pulses: puy and green lentils, chickpeas, split peas, soya beans, kidney, adzuki and haricot beans – one portion is 75–100g (2½–3½oz/½ cup) cooked.

Berries: blueberries, cherries, raspberries, blackberries and strawberries – one portion is 60–80g (2¼–2¾oz/½ cup).

Low glycaemic fruit: apples, pears, plums, peaches, nectarines and citrus fruits.

If you are having difficulty with your blood sugar restrict these foods in your diet initially:

CARBOHYDRATES TO RESTRICT
High-glycaemic fruits: melon (particularly watermelon), grapes, pineapple, mango, guava, lychees, raisins and banana.

CARBOHYDRATES TO AVOID COMPLETELY
All refined white flour and sugar, including breads, cereals, pasta, bagels, and pastries; sugar in all its forms and sweeteners, including high-fructose corn syrup (HFCS); dried fruit, fruit juice, soft drinks, sugary beverages, hot chocolate, coffee, tea and alcohol.

GI refers to the extent to which blood glucose rises after eating a food as compared to pure glucose, which is given a benchmark score of 100. A food's GI is influenced by its fibre, protein and fat content, as well as how it has been processed and/or cooked.

The GL of a food, however, is a more useful measure as this takes account of the GI and the amount eaten. A food's GL is calculated by multiplying its GI score by the amount of carbohydrate per serving. A GL of 15–20 or above is considered high and one of 10 or under is considered low.

Essentially foods that contain a higher proportion of carbohydrate tend to have a higher GL than foods that comprise more protein, fat, fibre or water. So meat, poultry, fish, eggs, beans, pulses, nuts, seeds, dairy, vegetables, fruits, fats and oils and whole grains have a lower GL than refined foods such as white starches, sugars and alcohol.

So if you are looking for minimal effect on blood-sugar levels opt for low-GL foods the majority of the time – see page 19 for a list of the best carbohydrates to include in your diet.

THE HIGHS AND LOWS OF BLOOD SUGAR

As a result of poor dietary choices blood-sugar levels can rise and fall rapidly through-out the day (*see* box, page 23). After you have a meal, drink or snack high in carbo-hydrates, your blood-glucose levels will soar. To compensate insulin will escort the glucose into cells to be used for energy and any excess will be dumped as fat. This can result in a crashing blood-glucose level and when blood sugar plummets, lethargy, sleepiness, irritability and cravings set in. It can also lead to anxiety, palpitations, head-

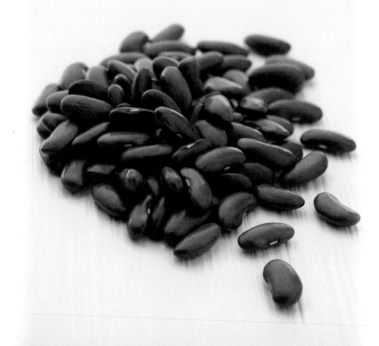

aches or light-headedness. These symptoms of low blood sugar prompt your body to react and start craving foods or drinks that will lift it again. This could include a cup of coffee or tea, a cola, a cigarette or a bar of chocolate. (Although coffee and cigarettes do not actually contain sugar, they stimulate the release of sugar stores in the body. Alcohol also raises blood-sugar levels only to send them plummeting again soon afterwards.) Meanwhile, your body is busy taking its own urgent steps in order to get blood-sugar levels back within the ideal parameters. It rapidly releases stores of glucose and, at the same time, pumps out adrenalin to make sure the fuel gets around the body as quickly as possible.

The problem is that the body's response is short lived and it leads to a vicious cycle resulting in more cravings and mood fluctuations and poorer concentration and reduced energy levels.

EATING TO BALANCE BLOOD SUGAR

Our diet has changed considerably over the last 30 to 50 years. One of the biggest changes is our increased sugar consumption and in particular consumption of high-fructose corn syrup (HFCS). This is commonly found in processed foods and sugary soft drinks. While all sugar is harmful our bodies deal with HFCS differently from other sugars. It is metabolized by the liver and triggers lipogenesis (the production of fats like triglycerides and cholesterol). This can increase our risk of cardiovascular disease and fatty liver. The glucose triggers spikes in insulin contributing to insulin resistance, diabetes and inflammation. This in turn can result in fluctuations in blood sugar, damage to brain cells and low energy levels.

Modern diets are also low in fibre and nutrients. Although food in Western countries may be readily available it is nutritionally poor. Fibre is important for balancing blood sugar as it slows down the absorption of sugar into the bloodstream. It also helps us feel fuller for longer so we are less likely to snack. Soluble fibre from our diet comes from plant foods (fruits and vegetables), nuts, seeds, beans and pulses, and whole grains. Processed refined foods are generally much lower in essential fibre. Our diet is also lacking in key nutrients known to be important for balancing insulin and blood sugar. These include vitamin D, chromium, magnesium, zinc, biotin, omega 3 fats and antioxidants. Details on these nutrients are listed in the tables on pages 17 and 181–3. If you are suffering from poor blood-sugar control, you may need to increase your intake of foods that are rich in these nutrients. Ensuring our bodies are optimally nourished will help keep blood-sugar levels balanced through the day.

To stabilize blood-sugar levels it is important you take the following steps:

* Avoid all forms of sugar – this includes agave, maple syrup, honey, molasses, brown and white sugar and sweeteners.
* Avoid all processed, refined foods – these are often high in HFCS and trans fats (*see* pages 42–3). These include ready meals and takeaways as well as white refined grains and flour products (e.g. rice, pasta, wraps, rolls, breads, pastries).
* Choose foods with a low glycaemic load (GL) (*see* pages 18–20), as they slow down the release of glucose into the bloodstream. These include: proteins (lean meat, poultry, fish and shellfish, eggs, low-fat dairy, nuts and seeds); foods high in soluble fibre (beans, pulses, vegetables); and lower-sugar, colourful fruits (berries, apples, pears, plums, peaches, cherries, citrus).
* Get the balance right. Every meal should be mainly vegetables – with some lean protein and healthy fat. Cover half of your plate with low-starch vegetables. On one quarter of your plate add some protein and on the other quarter either 50–60g (1¾–2¼oz/⅓ cup) cooked whole grains or 60g (2oz/½ cup) starchy vegetables such as sweet potato or sweetcorn.
* Never eat carbohydrates on their own. Combine carbs with protein and fat at each meal and snack. For example, eat an apple with a handful of nuts, or rye crackers with hummus.
* If you have a problem balancing your blood-sugar levels, are insulin resistant or diabetic, then starchy foods like potatoes and grains (even whole grains) are not recommended. Cutting right back on starchy carbs has been found to reduce insulin fluctuations. As carbohydrates are still found in vegetables and fruits it is recommended that you limit fruit intake to two pieces a day.
* Switch to olive oil (containing monounsaturated fatty acids) in dressings and low-temperature cooking. Olive oil may help reduce insulin resistance.
* Include omega 3 fatty acids daily. These help improve insulin sensitivity and reduce inflammation. Eat oily fish (herring, mackerel, salmon, trout, sardines) three times a week. Include walnuts, flax (linseeds), hemp, chia and pumpkin seeds and their oils.
* Add apple cider vinegar to dressings. Vinegar has been found to lower post-eating blood-glucose and insulin levels.

THE BLOOD-SUGAR SEESAW

The dotted yellow line in the diagram below represents normal, healthy fluctuations in blood-sugar levels that occur over a period of a few hours or a whole day, depending on your metabolism and diet.

The red line represents undesirable extreme rises and falls in blood-sugar levels caused by a diet that throws the body's natural equilibrium out of kilter. If you notice that you are suddenly feeling tired and low, struggling to concentrate and craving sweet, starchy food, you are probably experiencing a blood-sugar drop. A common reaction is to grab a sugary snack, which, combined with your body's own efforts to resolve the crisis (see pages 20–21), causes blood-sugar levels to rise sharply. You may briefly feel better, but this sudden rise is quickly followed by another dramatic fall and the whole cycle begins again. This may occur twice during the day – mid-morning and mid-afternoon are often marked by drops in blood-sugar levels, especially if your breakfast and lunch are composed mainly of fast-releasing foods (e.g. cornflakes, white bread, bananas etc) – or it may occur as often as once an hour, if you regularly snack on fast-releasing foods.

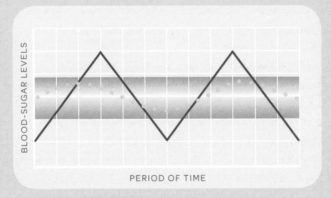

BLOOD-SUGAR LEVELS

PERIOD OF TIME

KEY

▬▬▬ ideal range of blood-sugar levels

• • • normal fluctuations in blood-sugar levels

▬▬▬ undesirable extreme fluctuations in blood-sugar levels

HOW TO EAT

◆ Eat little and often but do not overeat.

◆ You may find it easier to control your blood-glucose levels by eating little and often; that is, five small meals a day, rather than three large ones.

◆ Slow down. Take time to eat. Chew your food thoroughly and eat slowly as this reduces the body's glycaemic response to the meal.

NUTRITIONAL SUPPORT

In addition to eating low-GL foods, certain nutrients can actually enhance the processes that regulate blood-sugar levels. If you are showing signs of blood-sugar imbalances, then you may need to include some additional nutrients as supplements. A high-quality multivitamin formula may be a good place to start, but you may also benefit from specific nutrients such as the ones below. Always seek professional advice regarding the use of supplements especially if you are currently on medication.

Vitamin D3 improves metabolism influencing many different genes including those associated with diabetes. Vitamin D insufficiency is also commonplace. It is important to monitor your levels with your doctor to ensure it is at an optimal level.

Chromium is an important mineral for sugar metabolism and improving insulin sensitivity. The B vitamins, particularly biotin, are also involved in processing sugar, improving glucose metabolism.

Magnesium helps glucose enter the cells and helps convert glucose into energy.

Omega 3 fatty acids improve insulin sensitivity and lower cholesterol as well as reducing inflammation.

Alpha lipoic acid is a powerful antioxidant shown to reduce blood sugar and help prevent nerve damage and neuropathy (a nerve disorder associated with diabetes).

L-glutamine directly fuels the brain so can help reduce carbohydrate or sugar cravings.

Vanadium and *manganese* are minerals involved in the way the body handles glucose. Needed in very small amounts – normally found in a multivitamin formula.

Certain foods have been shown to balance blood-sugar levels. Cinnamon and catechins (found in green tea) are particularly beneficial. Just 1 teaspoon cinnamon can be effective in helping balance blood-sugar levels. Other helpful foods and herbal supplements include fenugreek seeds, bitter melon, gymnema leaf extract and aloe vera.

GOOD-MOOD SUMMARY

To optimize blood-sugar balance:

- base your meals around unprocessed whole foods
- avoid stimulants such as caffeine found in chocolate, coffee and tea
- avoid alcohol and cigarettes
- avoid sugar in all its forms, including sweeteners
- avoid refined, white and processed foods, ready meals and takeaways
- avoid fruit juice, squash, soft drinks and sugary beverages
- follow a low-glycaemic eating plan based around lean protein with some healthy fat and an abundance of low-glycaemic vegetables
- always eat carbohydrates with protein and healthy fat
- eat small meals/snacks five or six times a day
- include 1 teaspoon cinnamon daily and 4–6 cups green tea
- see pages 114–175 for some healthy recipe, meal and snack ideas
- consider taking nutritional supplements designed to support blood-sugar balance (*see* left)

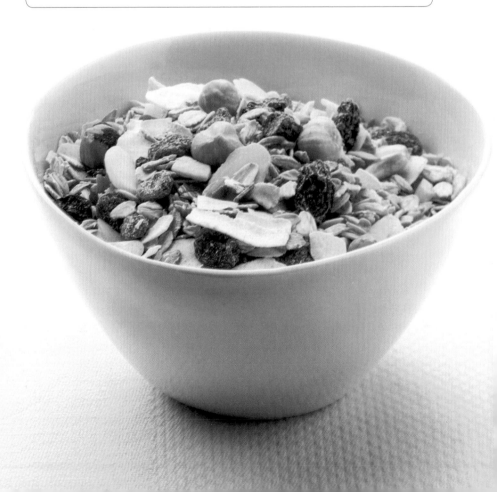

THE STRESS RESPONSE

While we all need a certain amount of stress to keep us motivated, when it takes over our lives it can adversely affect us.

Stress is defined as a real or imagined threat to our body. This can be emotional, physical or psychological. We all experience acute stressors and these are difficult to avoid. But this form of stress comes and goes. It is ongoing, unremitting stress that is more likely to affect our health, energy levels and mood.

The adrenal glands function as part of the hypothalamic–pituitary–adrenal (HPA) axis and control our response to stress. When we are under stress our adrenal glands produce the stress hormones adrenalin and cortisol. This accelerates many metabolic processes in our body – our breathing and heart rates increase, blood pressure rises and so does our blood sugar. The adrenals also release the hormone DHEA (dehydroepiandrosterone), which helps to maintain energy and counter the effects of cortisol. This is the initial "fight or flight" response and is designed to create short-term stimulation to help us cope with the stress experienced.

However, for many people the stress is not short lived – it continues, and ongoing stress demands further production of cortisol and DHEA. Chronically elevated cortisol has been shown to cause increased blood sugar and cholesterol, depression and even dementia. As the production of cortisol requires certain vitamins and minerals, ongoing high levels can deplete the body of key nutrients. Too much cortisol also interferes with thyroid and growth hormones and negatively affects our sleep patterns as well. Poor sleep has been linked to numerous health problems including fatigue, energy fluctuations, insulin resistance, low mood, poor cognitive function and depression. It can also aggravate existing conditions such as high blood pressure.

As stress becomes chronic our body's ability to cope is reduced. Gradually the production of cortisol and DHEA declines, we become depleted of key nutrients and energy levels plummet. In addition, as adrenalin is derived from the neurotransmitter dopamine (associated with motivation), demands to produce more and more stress hormones can lead to dopamine deficiency. This can result in low mood, apathy, depression and cravings for sugary-foods and caffeine.

BITE-SIZE SOLUTION

Drinking relaxing herbal teas, such as chamomile or lemon balm can help the body relax and unwind, whereas drinking caffeinated drinks like coffee has the opposite effect, putting more pressure on your body's stress-response mechanisms.

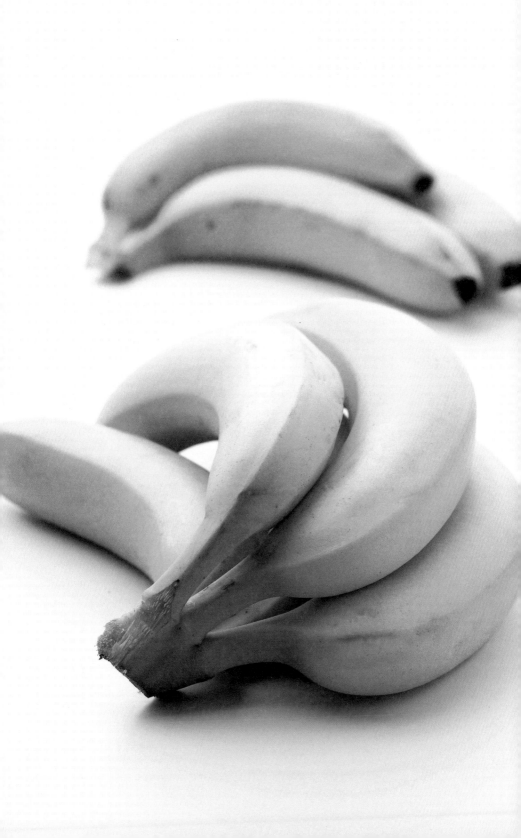

The following list highlights some of the signs and symptoms related to your current levels of stress. If you suspect stress is playing a role in your current health, seek support from a qualified nutritionist who can also arrange for an adrenal stress test to be undertaken.

SIGNS OF HIGH CORTISOL OUTPUT

* Tired but wired – you find it hard to unwind and relax
* Anxiety
* Negativity and depression
* Poor sleep
* Cravings for sugary and starchy foods or caffeine
* Irritability, on a "short fuse"
* Unable to deal with stressful situations
* Exhaustion on waking
* Weight gain around the abdomen

SIGNS OF LOW CORTISOL OUTPUT

* General fatigue
* Excessive sleep
* Fatigue, apathy
* Depression, tearfulness, SAD (seasonal affective disorder)
* Muscle and/or joint pains
* Poor memory, concentration and motivation

SUPPORTING YOUR STRESS RESPONSE THROUGH DIET

The effects of stress are shaped by our thoughts, attitudes and beliefs. While we may not be able to change all of our circumstances, we are able to change how we respond to the stressors. Stress management is therefore crucial to help you deal with ongoing stress in your life.

What and how we eat can also support our body's stress response. One of the first steps is to follow a strategy designed to balance your blood-sugar levels, as summarized on pages 16–25. When blood-sugar levels fall the adrenal glands are triggered to release adrenalin and then cortisol to help deal with the stress of perceived starvation. Cortisol induces glycogen breakdown in the liver, so that the bloodstream is replenished with glucose. So by taking action to stabilize blood sugar through the day you can avoid this additional stress on your adrenal glands.

NUTRIENTS FOR HEALTHY STRESS RESPONSE

To optimize the body's response to stress, we need a full range of nutrients, which is best obtained from a varied, balanced diet. The following nutrients are particularly important:

NUTRIENT	RICH FOOD SOURCES
Protein	Dairy products, eggs, fish, meat, poultry, soya
Vitamin B3	Beef liver, brewer's yeast, chicken, fish, sunflower seeds, turkey
Vitamin B5	Blue cheese, brewer's yeast, corn, eggs, lentils, liver, lobster, meats, peanuts, peas, soya beans, sunflower seeds, wheatgerm, whole-grain products
Vitamin B6	Avocados, bananas, bran, brewer's yeast, carrots, hazelnuts, lentils, rice, salmon, shrimps, soya beans, sunflower seeds, tuna, wheatgerm, whole-grain flour
Vitamin C	Blackcurrants, broccoli, Brussels sprouts, cabbage, grapefruit, guava, kale, lemons, oranges, papaya, peppers, potatoes, spinach, strawberries, tomatoes, watercress
Magnesium	Halibut, kelp, leafy green vegetables, nuts, squash, sunflower and pumpkin seeds
Omega 3 fatty acids	Herring, mackerel, wild salmon, sardines, trout, chia seeds, flaxseed, walnuts, pumpkin seeds

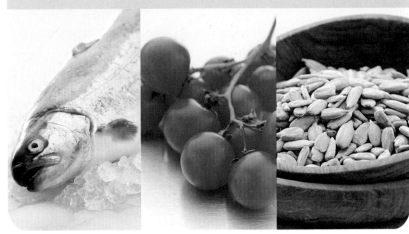

Regular protein is important, especially foods that contain tyrosine, which is the precursor to adrenalin and noradrenalin produced by the adrenal glands. Protein will also help balance your blood sugar. So include plenty of nuts, seeds, dairy products, fish, eggs and lean meat daily.

It is important to reduce your intake of adrenal stimulants such as sugars, refined carbohydrates, alcohol and excessive levels of caffeinated drinks (tea, coffee, cola) and foods (chocolate). Although coffee does have some health benefits, excessive caffeine intake can interfere with blood-sugar levels when you are under stress and decaffeinated hot drinks may be a better option. Green tea is also recommended, in moderation, because it contains L-theanine, which is thought to have a calming effect on the nervous system. In addition, green tea contains the chemical EGCG (epigallocatechin-3-gallate), a potent antioxidant that protects brain cells from damage. Recent studies

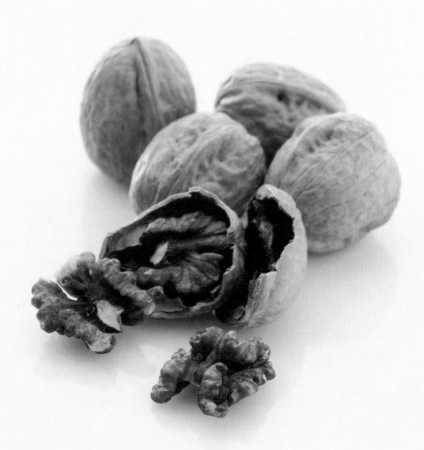

also indicate EGCG can improve cognitive function by promoting the generation of neuron cells, a process known as neurogenesis. Other calming herbal teas include chamomile and lemon balm.

NUTRIENTS AND HERBS FOR ADRENAL SUPPORT

In addition to a healthy diet that helps balance blood-sugar levels, there are certain nutrients (*see* table, page 29) and herbs that particularly nourish overworked adrenals. The key nutrients are magnesium, vitamin C and B vitamins. Magnesium deficiency has been linked to anxiety and poor sleep patterns. B vitamins, especially pantothenic acid (vitamin B5), are important for adrenal hormone production. Vitamin C is present in high concentrations in the adrenal glands and low levels will affect its function. You also need a good balance of essential fatty acids (EFAs), as these are crucial for the health of cell membranes where the receptors for adrenal hormones are located. Healthy cell membranes ensure that the substances that go in and out of each cell (for example, water, nutrients, hormonal messages and waste products) do so effectively. These fats also moderate the body's production of natural inflammatory substances, which in excess encourage the release of too much cortisol.

Certain herbs have been shown to help the body adapt to stress. These include licorice, rhodiola, ginseng and ashwagandha. Please seek advice from a qualified practitioner if considering herbal support. Maca (*Lepidium peruvianum*) is a Peruvian root that can be bought in powdered form from health food shops. It has long been used traditionally to support the body in times of stress and can easily be added to smoothies and desserts. It can also be used in baking.

EXERCISE, SLEEP AND STRESS MANAGEMENT

Exercise also plays a part in restoring the health of the adrenals, but in order to get the most benefit forget the mantra "no pain, no gain". Instead you should train within your limits, feeling comfortable and in control, and avoiding excessive strain. Many people who have fast-paced lives that exhaust their adrenals also follow a very rigorous exercise routine, not realizing that this too acts as a stressor. When you are run down, doing a hard workout at the gym is the last thing you need. Exercise itself increases levels of adrenalin and cortisol, which is partly why, when you have just finished the workout, you may feel particularly good. However, if you are suffering from adrenal burnout, this temporary high only exacerbates the problem.

If you are experiencing stress symptoms, it is important to balance exercises such as running, weight training, aerobics and cycling with more internal, meditative exercises such as gentle walking, qigong, Pilates, yoga and tai chi. These cultivate more energy than they expend enabling the body to recover and repair.

Rest and sleep are equally important to help support the adrenal glands. If you have trouble sleeping, make sure your bedroom is completely dark and well ventilated, switch off all the electrics and keep the two hours prior to bedtime free of computers, television, intense exercise, caffeine and bright lighting.

Finally, no dietary changes will restore your adrenal function to normal if you do not tackle the underlying sources of stress. This may involve reassessing your work, home or social life. If the stress is ongoing and you reach the stage where you feel you cannot cope, seek support. Talk to a sympathetic partner, friend, relative or colleague, or enlist the help of a life coach or professional counsellor (*see* page 187).

GOOD-MOOD SUMMARY

To improve your body's stress response:

* seek support from a qualified nutritionist who can organize an adrenal stress test to be undertaken to ascertain your current output of cortisol
* eat small meals or snacks five or six times a day, following the guidelines on pages 16–25 to balance blood sugar
* eat 1–2 tablespoons omega 3-rich seeds each day (e.g. flax, hemp, chia, sesame, pumpkin seeds)
* eat omega 3-rich oily fish two to three times a week (e.g. sardines, mackerel, trout, herring, salmon, kippers)
* avoid "stimulants", such as sugar and sugary foods or drinks, refined foods (including biscuits or white bread), coffee, tea, alcohol and cigarettes
* see pages 114–175 for a range of healthy recipe, meal and snack ideas
* take a blend of nutrients designed to support your adrenal glands (*see* page 29)
* incorporate appropriate exercise regularly – but listen to your body
* get enough sleep: if you are finding it hard to sleep well, discuss options with your healthcare practitioner
* make yourself part of a good social support network
* review stress in your life and make positive changes to reduce levels if needed

NUTRIENT SUPPLIES

Although the list of symptoms that can result from even a mild nutrient deficiency is seemingly endless, mood swings, irritability, tiredness and poor concentration are all classic signs that your brain, and the rest of your body, are not receiving all the nutrients they need.

Every single process and chemical reaction that takes place in your body depends on a regular supply of "micro" nutrients, such as vitamins and minerals, as well as "macro" nutrients, including protein, carbohydrates, fats and water, which we need in larger amounts. It makes sense, then, that the raw materials you feed your body affect the way it works, and therefore have an impact on your moods and energy levels.

NUTRIENTS FOR MOOD

For optimal brain health, we need healthy nerves and balanced levels of neurotransmitters (*see* pages 9–12) and blood sugar (*see* pages 16–25). Indeed, pretty much all the systems in our body need to be in good working order, even those governing our digestion and detoxification (*see* pages 44–51). Without a good supply of nutrients, these systems will not function as well as they could. Even slightly reduced levels of key nutrients can affect how we think and feel.

The table on page 36 lists the food sources of key nutrients for optimal brain function. For lowering homocysteine (*see* box, page 34) the key vitamins are folic acid, B6 and B12. Studies have shown that supplementation of folic acid at 800mcg (0.8mg) daily in people with slightly raised homocysteine improves memory and cognitive function.

B12 is a particularly important B vitamin as we age. This is because it becomes more difficult to absorb from food, likely to be related to decreasing levels of stomach acid. A deficiency can lead to pernicious anaemia. B12 deficiency is also more likely in vegans, as the main sources include meat, fish, eggs and dairy foods.

B6 not only helps lower homocysteine but is important in the production of the neurotransmitters dopamine and serotonin, making it useful for boosting mood and promoting sleep.

BITE-SIZE SOLUTION

Focus on the quality of the food you eat. This is more important than quantity or calories. By focusing on quality you will feel satisfied and avoid cravings, empty calories and foods that fail to nourish your body.

THE HOMOCYSTEINE CONNECTION

We have already seen that optimal brain health requires, among other things, the appropriate balance of neurotransmitters. For this your body needs to provide the right building blocks, normally amino acids, as well as support the effective conversion of these components into neurotransmitters. One of the most important processes involved in maintaining an optimal balance is methylation. This is a series of chemical reactions that help create and balance neurotransmitters, build cells and protect your brain from damage. Methylation is also involved in the processing of phospholipids, a type of fat that supports the neurotransmitter receptors and is found in the myelin sheath that protects cells. Some people are not particularly efficient at methylating, and one way we can assess this is by measuring the level of an amino acid in your blood known as homocysteine.

Homocysteine is naturally converted into the amino acid known as S-adenosyl methionine. This conversion requires a range of B vitamins, including B2, B6, B12 and folate, as well as magnesium, zinc and trimethylglycine (TMG). A high level of homocysteine has been shown to double your risk of depression. A high homocysteine level has also been linked to decline in cognitive function, dementia and Alzheimer's. You may be able to ask your healthcare practitioner to measure your homocysteine level or you can arrange for a private lab test through a qualified nutritionist. A low intake of these vitamins and minerals – particularly B vitamins – will lead to a raised level of homocysteine. In addition, a high intake of alcohol or caffeinated drinks, as well as smoking, can increase homocysteine levels.

A combination formula containing all the key nutrients for lowering homocysteine appears to be more effective than supplementing any one nutrient alone. As B vitamins and vitamin C are water-soluble, your body excretes them within a few hours of absorption. As a result, you'll need to eat food sources rich in these vitamins (*see* table, page 36) every day.

A zinc deficiency may be linked to depression, addiction problems, loss of appetite, low mood and energy. Mood and energy is often low as zinc is required for the production of thyroid and adrenal hormones. Low levels of zinc have also been associated with anorexia.

The mineral magnesium is vital if nerve cells (neurons) are to communicate effectively with one another and it is involved in many enzyme reactions in the body and brain including the production of neurotransmitters. It is depleted by stress and signs of deficiency can include anxiety, insomnia, muscle cramps, spasms and migraines.

Iron is important for the structure and function of the central nervous system. Cognitive and behavioural disorders in children may be linked to low iron intake. Low iron levels can also affect overall energy levels. The most easily absorbable form of iron is haem iron, which comes from lean red meat and the darker meat from game, poultry and oily fish, as well as from eggs. The body finds it more difficult to absorb vegetarian sources of iron (e.g. in beans, pulses, dried fruit, leafy green vegetables). For optimal absorption combine them with foods rich in vitamin C, such as fruit and raw or lightly cooked vegetables.

Essential fatty acids (EFAs) and phospholipids also play a crucial role in nerve messaging. See pages 42–3 for an explanation of how EFAs affect nerve cells and how to include more of the foods that are rich in EFAs in your diet.

Antioxidants play a protective role in optimal brain health. Deeply coloured fruits and vegetables are particularly rich sources, so aim to include a variety of these in your daily diet. Fruits and vegetables provide vitamins C and E and phytochemicals like flavonoids and carotenoids that help to protect the brain cells, neurotransmitters and the essential fats in the cell membranes from damage. Culinary herbs are also rich in phytonutrients, so include them liberally in cooking. Drink green tea too. High in anti-oxidants, it also contains an amino acid called L-theanine, which has been found to increase low levels of serotonin, dopamine and GABA, enhance learning and memory and reduce anxiety.

MAXIMIZING YOUR NUTRIENT INTAKE

With our busy lives many of us eat on the run, which can prevent us from digesting and absorbing our food well, or even choosing the most nutritious foods in the first place. To ensure that you are getting adequate nutrients from your diet, you need to follow some basic guidelines.

Highly processed, refined and overcooked foods are low in nutrients and often high in anti-nutrients and toxins meaning they can actually deplete our bodies of nutrients. Aim to eat as much fresh, unprocessed, unrefined food as possible. Ideally choose organic, local and seasonal produce.

Be careful not to overcook food, as heat destroys valuable nutrients – try to steam or quickly stir-fry vegetables, for example, and enjoy eating them "crunchy", rather than boiling them until they are soft. Include more raw vegetables and fruits in your diet. Try to include a raw mixed salad daily. It is also important to eat a variety of foods to ensure that you are getting the full spectrum of required nutrients. Even the healthiest food, if eaten repeatedly, may leave you short of the nutrients it does not contain.

BARE ESSENTIALS FOR OPTIMAL BRAIN FUNCTION

	ROLE	NUTRIENTS NEEDED	KEY FOODS
Serotonin	Feel-good neurotransmitter. Needed for good moods, healthy sleep patterns and appetite control. Derived from tryptophan.	Vitamins B3, B6, biotin, folic acid, zinc	Eggs, soy foods, spirulina, fish, cheese, pumpkin and sesame seeds, beans and pulses, game and red meat
Dopamine	Stimulating neurotransmitter. Needed for feeling motivation and pleasure. Derived from amino acids tyrosine or its precursor phenylalanine.	Vitamins B3, B6, B12, C, copper, folic acid, iron, magnesium, manganese, zinc	Eggs, soy foods, spirulina, poultry, dairy, fish and seeds (pumpkin and sesame).
Acetylcholine	Neurotransmitter associated with memory and cognitive function. Requires choline. Choline is also an essential component of the neuron membranes (see below).	Vitamins B5, B1, B12, C, acetyl-L-carnitine (helps make acetylcholine and acts as an antioxidant)	Egg yolk, fish roe, liver (and other organ meats) and lecithin granules from health shops.
Healthy neurons	Nerve cells required for general health and to transmit messages efficiently.	Antioxidants, B vitamins, calcium, essential fatty acids, folic acid, magnesium, choline	Eggs, oily fish, lecithin granules, beef
Even blood-sugar levels	Dives in blood sugar send mood, energy and concentration crashing.	B vitamins, zinc, chromium, omega 3 fats, magnesium, vanadium, vitamin D, alpha lipoic acid, manganese	Lean meat, nuts, seeds, oily fish, leafy green vegetables, seafood, mushrooms

IS A "BALANCED" DIET ENOUGH?

Sadly, eating fresh, unprocessed food will not guarantee that your body gets all the nutrients it needs. The balanced-diet argument is partly based on the notion that our soils are rich in minerals that are absorbed by the plants growing in them, which we subsequently eat. Yet with today's intensive farming methods and artificial fertilizers, plants no longer need naturally mineral-rich soil to grow into the bumper-crop, over-sized, uniform fruits and vegetables we now expect to see on our supermarket shelves. Also, we do not always eat fruit and vegetables in season – many have been picked before they are ripe, stored for long periods of time and shipped across the world, none of which does their nutrient content much good.

The deficit of nutrients in our food is not the only factor that can leave us low in essential goodness. We are also exposed to many "anti-nutrients" – substances that deplete our stock of nutrients when they are processed in our bodies. Fizzy drinks, sugar, coffee, tea, alcohol and cigarettes interfere with our body's ability to absorb minerals. Overcooked (charred or blackened) meat contains chemicals that can encourage the production of potentially carcinogenic compounds and cause oxidative stress and damage to cells. By dramatically reducing your consumption of these substances, you can boost your body's intake of vital health- and mood-enhancing nutrients.

For a list of other foods that are rich in many of the nutrients mentioned in the table opposite, see the table on pages 180–183. If you are worried that you may be lacking in certain nutrients, you should see a qualified nutritionist, who will be able to carry out tests and suggest improvements to your diet to overcome any deficiencies.

GOOD-MOOD SUMMARY

To maximize your nutrient levels:

* eat fresh, seasonal, preferably organic whole foods
* include a variety of deeply coloured fruit and vegetables daily
* eat foods that have not been highly refined or processed
* reduce your intake of "anti-nutrients": alcohol, coffee, tea, fizzy drinks, sugar, fried food, foods containing trans fats (e.g. margarine and manufactured sauces and salad dressings)
* avoid blackened, burnt meat or fish
* avoid recreational drugs as well as nicotine, alcohol, caffeine
* see pages 114–175 for healthy recipe, meal and snack ideas
* consider a homocysteine test to check B-vitamin levels and methylation
* for a full assessment of your nutrient status, visit a nutritionist who will be able to give you guidance on your individual requirements

HEALTHY FATS

Many people assume that all fat is bad for them. However, some fats – particularly essential fatty acids – are not only healthy, but play a vital role in brain function. As well as helping the brain function better, some of them are used to build the brain and protect it from degeneration. Increasing your intake of these "good" fats and eating less of the "bad" fats can have a noticeable impact on your moods.

On the list below, tick any of the symptoms that you experience regularly:

- ☐ dry skin, itchy skin
- ☐ acne
- ☐ asthma
- ☐ dermatitis
- ☐ eczema
- ☐ psoriasis
- ☐ cracked/brittle nails
- ☐ dry, limp hair, dry scalp
- ☐ aching joints/arthritis
- ☐ depression
- ☐ aggression
- ☐ low mood
- ☐ anxiety

If you regularly suffer from the above signs and symptoms, your diet may be lacking in omega 3 and omega 6 fats, the two families of essential fatty acids (EFAs).

TYPES OF FATS

The types of fat that we eat have a considerable impact on our health. There are three main types of dietary fat (also known as lipids): triglycerides, phospholipids and sterols (such as cholesterol).

BITE-SIZE SOLUTION

If you're a vegetarian or vegan, or you don't like fish, it is particularly important you consume plenty of flax, chia and hemp seeds and their oils. These are all useful sources of omega 3 fats. Aim for 2–3 tablespoons daily and consider taking an omega 3 supplement as well as a multivitamin to ensure effective conversion.

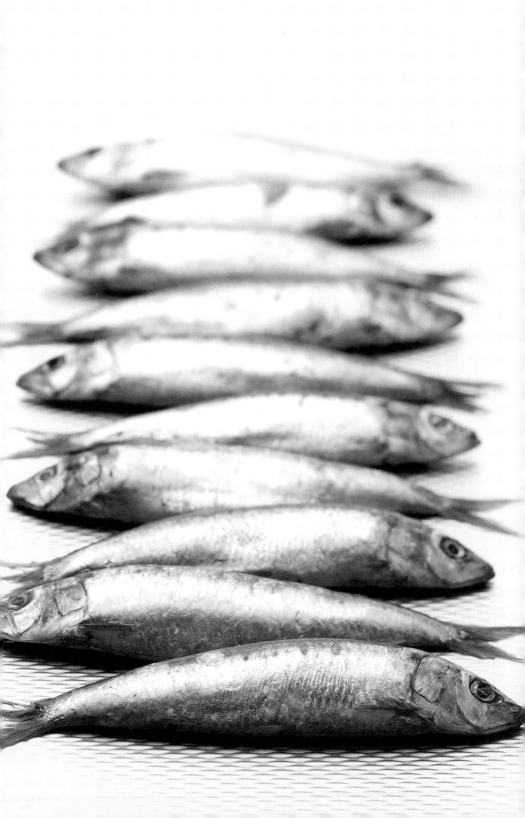

Most body fats and almost all the fats we eat are triglycerides, the most common type of fat. Triglycerides can be either saturated or unsaturated, which refers to their chemical structure. Saturated fats – those mainly found in animal products such as meat and dairy foods, as well as in coconut – are useful for cooking as they are more stable and less prone to damage than unsaturated fats. The long-held view that saturated fats are a primary cause of chronic cardiovascular diseases is now being challenged: the incidence of such conditions has been rising despite the replacement of much dietary animal fat with higher levels of starches and vegetable fats. Saturated fats will only increase levels of harmful LDL cholesterol and triglycerides when eaten in excess.

Coconut oil (see box, opposite) appears to be a healthier saturated fat because, although it can raise harmful LDL cholesterol if you eat it in excess, in small amounts it appears to raise protective HDL cholesterol. It also contains medium-chain triglycerides (MCTs), which are preferentially burnt by the body for energy rather than being stored as fat. It also contains the fatty acid lauric acid, which our bodies convert into a compound called monolaurin, which may help support the immune system. Other beneficial fatty acids found in animal fats include capric and caprylic acids, which have anti-microbial properties.

Unsaturated fats can be further subdivided into monounsaturated and polyunsaturated fats. Examples of rich sources of monounsaturated fat include olive oil (see box, opposite), rapeseed oil, rice bran oil, as well as avocados and most nuts. Polyunsaturated fats are also known as essential fatty acids (see below).

Unsaturated fats perform vital structural and functional jobs in the body; for example, they are an important component of cell membranes including those of brain cells. When choosing meat and dairy products, opt for organic, grass-fed varieties, as a greater proportion of their fat content is unsaturated.

ESSENTIAL FATTY ACIDS (EFAs)

All natural fatty acids can be synthesized in the human body except for essential fatty acids (EFAs), which can only be obtained through what we eat. EFAs are converted in the body (with the help of certain vitamins and minerals) into more concentrated versions of the fats and other substances. These are put to very good use in balancing hormones, keeping skin smooth and soft, improving hair and nail growth – and more. However, it is the role of the EFAs in ensuring that brain cells and neurotransmitters work efficiently that makes them such an important factor in maintaining stable moods and optimum brain power.

OILS FOR COOKING

Despite their bad press saturated fats are useful for cooking because they are the most stable fat and thus the least likely to become damaged by oxidation. For example, if you are going to roast or stir-fry vegetables it would be healthier to use coconut oil in small quantities than to use a vegetable oil. For this reason coconut oil has been used in recipes in this book. As coconut oil is expensive, olive oil could be used as an alternative, but it is better to use olive oil at a lower temperature. When choosing olive oil, choose one that is organic, virgin, and cold pressed. Like olive oil, rapeseed oil is a good source of monounsaturated fat, but because it also contains omega 3 it is more prone to damage if heated to high temperatures.

There are two families of EFAs: omega 3 and omega 6. Omega 6 essential fatty acids are found in vegetable oils, such as sunflower, and sesame and pumpkin seeds and their oils. Evening primrose oil and borage oil contain forms of an important omega 6 fat called gamma linolenic acid (GLA). You should include in your daily diet foods containing natural omega 6 fats such as raw seeds, especially sunflower, pumpkin, chia, sesame and hemp seeds, and their oils. Nuts also contain omega 6 fats. Always choose raw, unsalted nuts and seeds.

Omega 3 essential fatty acids are found in pumpkin, chia and hemp seeds, walnuts and flaxseed oil, as well as cold-water oily fish such as mackerel, herring, pilchards, sardines, salmon and fresh tuna.

As seeds are a wonderful source of these omega 3 fats as well as protein, vitamins and minerals it is recommended that you consume at least 1 tablespoon of seeds daily or their oils.

Ensure that the oils you buy are organic and cold pressed and keep them in the fridge. It is best not to heat them, as this can damage the delicate fatty acids.

In addition you should aim to eat two or three portions of oily fish a week. If you are pregnant or breastfeeding, this should be reduced to one or two portions per week, owing to the concern about possible contamination with methylmercury, dioxins and polychlorinated biphenyls. The most polluted fish are the larger varieties like shark, swordfish, marlin and tuna and these should be avoided, especially during pregnancy.

As well as eating foods rich in these omega fats, you should also include foods containing the nutrient co-factors for the enzymes used in the conversion of the essential fats to the active forms known as EPA (eicosapentaenoic acid), DHA (docosahexaenoic acid) and GLA. Your body and brain will only benefit fully from all those nuts, seeds and oily fish if this conversion takes place. Key co-factor nutrients include magnesium, zinc, B vitamins, biotin and vitamin C. Aim to increase your intake of leafy green vegetables, lean meat and fish, nuts, seeds and make sure you eat two or three portions of fruit daily.

HEALTHY FATS IN A HEALTHY BALANCE

Nutritionists advise that approximately 30% of your diet should be made up of fat. The majority of this should be in the form of monounsaturated fat. It is also recommended you eat foods rich in the essential omega 3 and 6 fats.

In today's typical diet, it is common to have a higher intake of omega 6 fats than omega 3, yet for optimum health and stable moods, you need to achieve a balance between the two. An excessive intake of omega 6 fats compared to omega 3 fats has been linked to inflammation. The recipes on pages 114–175 give inspiring suggestions for boosting your omega 3 intake if it is trailing behind.

BRAIN FOOD

Essential fatty acids are required for the production of phospholipids, which as we have seen, are a vital part of the receptors of brain cells for neurotransmitter function and also form part of the protective myelin sheath around the neurons. If you are lacking in these essential fats or if you are eating much more omega 6 than omega 3 fats, this can affect neurotransmitter signalling. EFA deficiency is linked to cognitive and mood disorders including depression, and improving the levels and/or ratios of omega 3 and omega 6 fats can help treat these symptoms.

One kind of phospholipid called phosphatidyl choline (PC) is the building block for the neurotransmitter acetylcholine, vital for memory (*see* pages 10–11). Key food sources of PC include fish, beef and eggs. You can also take a supplement called lecithin in the form of granules or capsules. The granules can be sprinkled over food or added to smoothies.

Another type of phospholipid found in fish is phosphatidyl serine (PS). This is highly concentrated in the brain and can aid cognitive function including memory, alertness and concentration. It can also be useful in combating the effects of stress.

HYDROGENATED FATS AND TRANS FATS

The problem with essential fatty acids is that they are very sensitive to damage from a combustion process called oxidation, which can transform them into what are known as hydrogenated or trans fats. This slight change has dramatic effects on the way in which the fat can be used in the body and ultimately on our health, including our moods and memory. Hydrogenated and trans fats have been linked to cardiovascular disease and may affect brain function by adversely influencing cell health.

To extend their shelf life, many processed oils and margarines have been heated and treated, forming trans fats; many convenience foods, especially baked goods, sauces and salad dressings, also contain them. Try to avoid sources of trans fats in your diet. The best way to do this is to cut out all processed foods that contain vegetable fats or other oils from plant sources (except coconut or palm oils), unless they are clearly stated to be "unhydrogenated". Store cold-pressed oils and fresh seeds in the fridge, where they are protected from rancidity caused by heat, light and oxygen exposure.

Antioxidant nutrients, such as vitamins A, C and E, selenium, sulphur and zinc, provide further protection for the essential fats in your body, so it is important to include plenty of antioxidant-rich foods in your diet (*see* table, page 181). Eat a wide range of brightly and deeply coloured fruits and vegetables daily. Antioxidants that help prevent lipid peroxidation are alpha lipoic acid (made in the body but some is found in beef, liver and dark green leafy vegetables), vitamin E (found in wheatgerm, seeds and avocado) and CoQ10 (made by the body).

GOOD-MOOD SUMMARY

To optimize your body's supply and balance of essential fats:

- use cold-pressed, unrefined seed oil (e.g. flaxseed) on salads, stirred into soups, on porridge or added to smoothies
- grind a blend of raw pumpkin, sesame, chia, flax and hemp seeds and consume 1 tablespoon daily
- snack on nuts and seeds or use them sprinkled on cereal or salads
- eat cold-water oily fish (such as salmon, mackerel, sardines, trout and herring) two or three times a week
- eat choline-rich foods such as eggs regularly and also consider taking a lecithin supplement daily
- use coconut oil for high-temperature cooking or olive oil at lower temperatures
- when eating meat and dairy products, opt for organic, grass-fed varieties
- avoid all refined, processed oils, including the processed foods that contain them
- limit your intake of fried foods – bake, poach or steam instead
- eat plenty of fresh fruit and vegetables daily to maximize your intake of antioxidants
- drink green tea daily (3–5 cups) for additional antioxidant protection

NATURAL DETOXIFICATION

How you think and feel is, to a large extent, dictated by how well your body is digesting and assimilating food, absorbing nutrients, detoxifying and eliminating waste. Although your brain may seem a long way from your gut, liver and bowels, it relies on them in order to function effectively.

On a day-to-day basis our normal body processes produce an array of compounds (hormones, neurotransmitters, and so on), all of which need to be safely deactivated and eliminated once they have done their job. This is in addition to the food, drinks and medications we may consume and exposure to toxins from our environment such as air pollution and cigarette smoke.

Our body's detoxification system includes the liver, the gastro-intestinal tract, the skin, the lungs and the kidneys. These organs help to process and transform toxins so they can be safely eliminated from the body. If these body systems are not working optimally then potentially our toxic load increases and we can experience a range of signs and symptoms. These include the following:

* headaches
* night sweats
* fatigue and sluggishness
* skin eruptions/spots
* low mood and irritability
* poor cognition/foggy head
* chemical, odour or pollution sensitivities, such as sneezing and/or dermatitis
* poor tolerance to alcohol
* adverse reactions to foods and/or food additives
* bloating, excess wind and constipation
* chronic itching/hives/rashes
* excessive mucus or sinus problems
* bitter taste in the mouth
* coffee leaves you feeling jittery or unwell

BITE-SIZE SOLUTION

Looking to lose weight? Then it's worth knowing that toxins interfere with and slow down your metabolism contributing to weight gain and blood-sugar imbalances. Keeping your diet clean and unprocessed may help you shed the pounds.

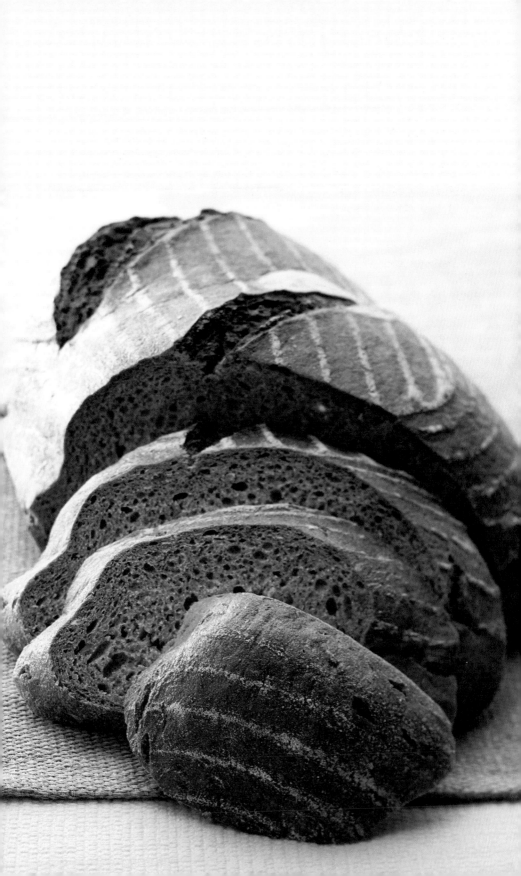

If you are experiencing some of the symptoms above you are likely to benefit from improving your detoxification potential. Your liver is the central clearing-house of your body and has an incredibly important impact on your health. However, there is also a direct link between gut health and liver function. So it is important your digestion is working optimally. This may help to minimize the production and movement of toxins across the gut membrane into the bloodstream.

OPTIMIZING DIGESTION

Digestive imbalances are often a contributing factor to many ongoing health conditions including low mood and energy levels. Therefore, in addition to detoxification it is important to optimize your digestive health too. This includes producing sufficient stomach acid and digestive enzymes to help break down food, maintaining a healthy gut membrane and gut flora for optimum absorption of nutrients, as well as promoting effective elimination of waste material.

The reason why digestive health is so important to how we think and feel is that the gastro-intestinal tract is connected to the central nervous system (CNS) via the enteric nervous system, also known as the gut–brain axis. In fact the gut is sometimes referred to as a neurological organ. Studies have shown that bloating and other gut symptoms can be linked to depression, anxiety and stress. In turn this can affect not only how well your gut functions but how you feel (*see* pages 56–7).

A compromised digestion can often result in intestinal permeability (sometimes referred to as "leaky gut"), where the gut wall becomes damaged allowing bacteria and undigested food to escape into the body. This can allow undigested proteins to enter the bloodstream through the gut wall causing food reactions and increasing the toxic burden on the body. This can result in inflammatory processes and immune reactions which can disturb the balance of neurotransmitters in the brain. An increase in toxic load also leads to further oxidative damage and inflammation, which places additional demands on the liver and increases our body's requirement for vitamins, minerals and antioxidants – the same nutrients required for efficient production and transmission of neurotransmitters.

BITE-SIZE SOLUTION

Eating foods that are rich in soluble fibre aids elimination of toxins. Good food sources include vegetables, beans, pulses, flaxseed, chia seed, oats, brown rice, and fresh and dried fruit. Many of the recipes in this book contain foods rich in soluble fibre.

BURDENING THE SYSTEM

What we eat has changed dramatically over the last 50 years or so. Today's highly processed, high-sugar, high-fat, low-fibre diet is low in essential nutrients, yet high in chemicals and toxins that will injure the gut, alter our gut flora and increase toxic load. An imbalance in our gut flora can lead to compromised detoxification processes, which in turn causes an increased oxidative load and then inflammation.

Our highly stressed lifestyles also influence our digestive health. When we are under stress our digestive system shuts down, resulting in symptoms such as nausea, indigestion, bloating, constipation and abdominal pain.

TOXIC EXPOSURE

The extent to which toxins affect our health depends not only on how well our detoxification systems are functioning but also on our level of exposure to toxins. Therefore, it is important you take steps to adapt your lifestyle and diet to reduce your exposure. Aim to make the following changes:

- Reduce your exposure to environmental pollutants, at home, at work and outdoors.
- Look for hair care and skin care products without added alcohol, sodium lauryl sulphate, paraben, phthalate or other petrochemicals. Avoid antiperspirants and antacids that contain aluminium and purchase natural cleaning products.
- Reduce or stop smoking and use of recreational drugs.
- Discuss your current medication with your healthcare practitioner.
- Keep active – any exercise that promotes sweating can help detoxification. Similarly, traditional and infrared saunas and magnesium sulphate baths (Epsom Salts) can stimulate elimination of toxins.
- Avoid eating larger oily fish such as shark, marlin, tuna and swordfish. These are likely to be more highly contaminated with pollutants such as methylmercury.
- Filter tap water with a multi-stage carbon filter or reverse-osmosis filter.
- Minimize your intake of bottled water in soft plastic containers, as chemicals from the plastics often leach into the water.
- Avoid sipping your takeaway hot drink through the plastic lid. Similarly, avoid using plastics in the microwave and check that containers used for food storage and smoothie shakers are free from the chemical bisphenol A (BPA).
- Switch from plastic, non-stick or aluminium cookware to glass, iron or ceramic alternatives and try not to use cling film or aluminium foil.
- Minimize your exposure to low-level electromagnetic fields by restricting your mobile phone use and limiting the amount of electrical equipment in the bedroom.

SUPPORTING DETOXIFICATION NATURALLY

If you are concerned about your toxic load, be wary of detoxification products and diets. You may have read about 48-hour detox fasts designed to ease the strain on the liver, but these can be counter-productive. During a fast, as the body's storage of fat is broken down, toxins can be released from fat cells into the bloodstream, which actually places an additional burden on the liver rather than giving it a break. For effective detoxification your body requires protein and key nutrients. When you go on a fast, you deplete these nutrients, which can result in a range of symptoms such as headaches, nausea, muscle aches, low mood and fatigue.

To optimize detoxification, keep your diet as clean and as unprocessed as possible. You will also need to avoid substances that give your liver a hard time. For natural detoxification support follow these guidelines:

WHAT TO EAT

* Where possible choose organic foods to minimize exposure to pesticides, antibiotics and additives.
* Include a wide range of brightly coloured fruits, vegetables and herbs rich in antioxidants, which can support the detoxification pathways and protect the body from oxidative damage.
* Certain foods are known to support liver detoxification, so include these daily. They include cruciferous vegetables (e.g. broccoli, kale, cauliflower, cabbage, pak choi and watercress), berries, green tea, herbs such as coriander and parsley, onions and garlic, beetroot and turmeric.
* Include foods rich in essential fats (*see* pages 40–41) and vitamin E (nuts, seeds, and avocado).
* Include high-quality protein foods daily – these are essential for the liver detoxification pathways. Good sources include lean meat, fish, eggs, poultry and game.
* Support your digestion by including probiotics such as natural live yogurt, kefir and miso. You may also wish to consider a probiotic supplement. Include foods that contain digestive enzymes, such as pineapple, which contains bromelain, and papaya.
* Stay regular. A daily bowel movement will help eliminate toxins. One of the most effective ways to avoid constipation is to take 1–2 tablespoons ground flaxseed daily with a large glass of water. Also include plenty of soluble fibre in your daily diet.
* Keep hydrated. As well as helping to stave off constipation, drinking at least 1l (35fl oz/4 cups) water daily will dilute toxins in the blood. It is best to drink filtered water and include herbal, green tea, green juices and green smoothies too.

KEY NUTRIENTS FOR LIVER DETOXIFICATION

PHASE 1

NUTRIENT	RICH FOOD SOURCES
Glutathione	Onions, garlic
Coenzyme Q10	Oily fish, spinach, seeds, nuts
Vitamin C	Broccoli, pepper, citrus fruits, berries
Vitamin E	Seeds, nuts, avocado
Selenium	Seeds, nuts, fish
Beta-carotene	Carrots, watermelon, sweet potato, butternut squash, pumpkin, apricots
Omega 3 fats	Flax, chia, hemp seeds, cold-water oily fish (sardines, mackerel, trout, herring, anchovies, salmon)
Phytonutrients	Berries, red onions, green tea, turmeric, culinary herbs
Glucosinolates	Cruciferous vegetables (broccoli, cabbage, kale, spinach, pak choi, watercress, cauliflower)

PHASE 2

PATHWAY	BENEFICIAL FOODS
Glucoronidation	Apples, Brussels sprouts, cabbage, broccoli
Glycine and glutamine conjugation	Sprouted beans, Brussels sprouts, root vegetables (swede, parsnip, carrot, beetroot)
Glutathione conjugation	Onions, garlic
Sulphation	Eggs, meat, fish, game, poultry, beans, onions, garlic
Methylation	Leafy greens, lean meat, eggs, root vegetables, beans, pulses

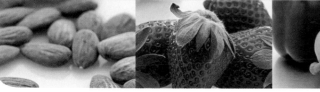
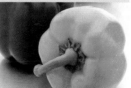

WHAT TO AVOID

- Caffeine and alcohol.
- High-sugar or high-salt processed foods and drinks.
- Fried foods, burnt meat and processed meats high in preservatives.
- Damaged fats: oxidized, hydrogenated or trans fats – often found in processed foods, ready meals and takeaways.
- Reduce the intake of saturated fat (full-fat dairy and fatty meat products).
- If you have a sensitive digestion consider avoiding gluten grains – wheat, barley, rye, and spelt.
- Eliminate known allergen foods from your diet (*see* page 57), as these place additional stress on your digestive health.

HOW YOUR LIVER DETOXIFIES

Potentially harmful substances are detoxified by the liver in two distinct phases, often termed phase 1 and phase 2. Your liver detoxification capacity depends partly on factors you cannot do anything about such as your genes, age and gender, but it is also strongly influenced by your diet and lifestyle.

These two phases combine to transform toxins into water-soluble compounds so that they can be safely eliminated. In phase 1 (often referred to as "oxidation"), enzymes convert the toxins into a form that can be disarmed, but in doing so they can produce potentially more reactive and toxic intermediates. To neutralize their toxicity, these reactive intermediates are acted on in phase 2 (known as "conjugation") through a range of chemical pathways. The five main ones are glucoronidation, glycine and glutamine conjugation, glutathione conjugation, sulphation and methylation. All of these pathways require key nutrients and dietary amino acids (from protein foods).

Normally, the two phases operate in harmony. However, when your body has a higher than normal toxic exposure phase 1 can accelerate and phase 2 may struggle to keep up, which can lead to a build up of toxic intermediates. This can cause tissue damage leading to inflammation and degenerative diseases. Therefore, it is important that you include a wide range of nutrients to support both phases.

GOOD-MOOD SUMMARY

To optimize your digestion and detoxification:

- include plenty of antioxidant-rich fruits and vegetables daily – preferably eat them raw or lightly steamed
- eat onion, garlic and eggs rich in sulphur compounds for liver function
- choose clean, unprocessed whole foods, limiting sugar and refined carbohydrates – focus on organic meats, eggs, fish, fruits and vegetables, whole grains, beans, pulses, nuts and seeds and olive oil
- include foods rich in liver-supporting nutrients
- drink green and herbal teas and at least 1l (35fl oz/4 cups) filtered water daily
- reduce your exposure to environmental toxins
- avoid refined, processed foods, ready meals and takeaways
- avoid alcohol and caffeine
- keep your gut healthy – consider probiotic foods and supplements (*see* page 48)

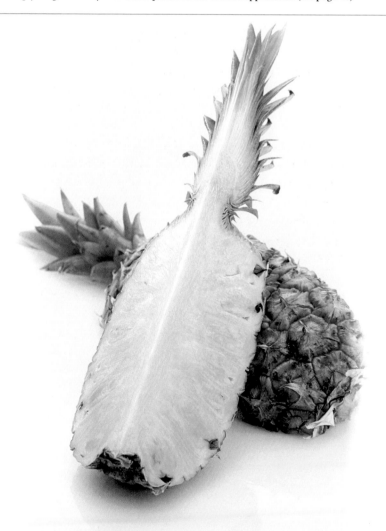

YOUR 7-DAY CLEANSE

If you feel your body needs a kick-start cleanse then consider undertaking this 7-day detox. You should then aim to keep toxic load to a minimum by following the recommendations on page 47. A cleansing week can be particularly useful to help break unhelpful eating patterns and nourish your liver and digestive systems so that they function more efficiently. It can be a useful way to restore energy levels – both mental and physical. Please note that such a programme should not be undertaken if you are suffering from any long-term health condition, are pregnant or are on medication. If you are in any doubt, seek advice from your health practitioner.

THE WEEK BEFORE

Gradually start reducing your intake of tea, coffee, alcohol and sugar as well as processed foods. This reduces the risk of side effects such as headaches or muscle aches during the cleansing week.

Use this time to stock up on the food you need for the week and clear unhealthy processed foods out of your cupboards. This is not a fast but a light, cleansing programme designed to give natural support to your detoxification system.

Each day include the following:
- a large cup of hot water with the juice of a lemon to start the day
- at least 6 glasses of filtered water
- 1 tablespoon ground flaxseed or 1–2 teaspoons psyllium husks with a glass of water or green juice (*see* page 55)
- 2–3 green juices or green smoothies (*see* page 55)
- herbal teas (if you wish) throughout the day
- 15 minutes of gentle exercise morning and afternoon
- body brushing in the morning and an Epsom salt bath in the evening (*see* opposite)
- for lunch, a large raw mixed salad with some light protein (e.g. hummus, beans, etc)
- for dinner, a portion of lean protein (fish, poultry, beans, sprouted seeds, eggs) with lightly steamed or raw vegetables

Avoid the following:
- any foods to which you know you are allergic
- gluten foods such as wheat, barley, rye and spelt

- dairy foods and soya except for natural low-fat yogurt
- caffeine – coffee, tea and chocolate
- carbonated soft drinks, fruit juices, squash/cordial
- alcohol
- refined carbohydrates (sugary foods, white grains – bread, pasta, rice)
- foods containing trans fats and hydrogenated fats
- red meat and processed meat products
- salt

In addition to your juices, smoothies, lunch and dinner you may need to include one or two snacks to avoid feeling hungry. It is important to listen to your appetite and only eat if you really feel hunger pangs. Here are some healthy snack ideas:

- vegetable sticks with hummus or nut butter
- half an avocado
- handful of nuts or seeds
- hard-boiled egg
- miso soup
- marinated artichoke hearts
- handful of olives

SUPPORTIVE TREATMENTS

To get the most out of your cleansing week try to include one or more of these treatments or techniques daily:

Body brushing. This stimulates your lymphatic system and improves your circulation. Use a long-handled natural bristle brush and move it in long strokes toward your heart. Shower once you have finished.

Epsom salt bath. Magnesium sulphate crystals (commonly known as Epsom Salts) provide your body with sulphur and magnesium, which are important for detoxification pathways. Pour 2 cups into a warm bath and treat yourself to a 20-minute soak. This helps eliminate toxins from your body.

Sauna or steam. Heat encourages your body to sweat out impurities. Try and sweat for at least 10–15 minutes then have a cool shower. Repeat this, if you wish. Always drink plenty of water before and after a sauna or steam. Infrared saunas work at a lower temperature but can be more effective and better tolerated than regular saunas.

Sleep. Good sleep is essential for recovery and repair so make sure you get adequate sleep and if you feel tired go to bed early.

SUPPLEMENTS TO SUPPORT THE LIVER

To support your liver's ability to detoxify, consider taking certain supplements in addition to dietary changes. Always seek support from a qualified nutritionist regarding the use of supplements especially if you have any health conditions or are on any medication.

Your primary supplement should be a combination of digestive enzymes, probiotics and L-glutamine powder. This will help you digest food optimally, restore the balance of healthy bacteria in the gut and support the health of your gut lining. Then consider adding in the following:

N-acetyl cysteine (NAC). This amino acid increases glutathione, which is important for detoxification pathways. Take 600mg twice a day.

Milk thistle. Known to boost glutathione levels, this herb has long been used to treat liver conditions. Take 175mg of a standardized extract twice a day.

Buffered ascorbic acid (vitamin C). Take 1000mg twice daily, once with breakfast and once with dinner. Too much can cause diarrhoea so cut down if you experience this side effect.

MEAL PLANNING

For balanced and healthy recipe ideas, see pages 114–175. Here is an example of how a typical day's menu might look:

On waking: large glass of hot water and juice of ½ lemon
BREAKFAST: green juice or smoothie
SNACK: ½ avocado; green smoothie or juice
LUNCH: large raw salad with ½ can of beans or 1–2 boiled eggs
SNACK: vegetable sticks with nut butter; green smoothie or juice
DINNER: Roasted vegetables with steamed fish
Water throughout the day

CLEANSING RECIPES

Each recipe makes 1 large glass. You can make up a batch for the whole day and store covered in the fridge or, for optimum freshness, make when needed.

GREEN JUICES

Parsley cleanser
Juice 2 celery sticks with a bunch of parsley, 2 apples and 1 lemon.

Kale and apple greens
Juice 2–3 handfuls of kale, 2 apples and ½ cucumber.

Cucumber and ginger cleanse
Juice ½ lemon with 1 cucumber, a piece of fresh ginger and 1 pear.

GREEN SMOOTHIES

Mango greens
Blend together 1 ripe mango with a handful of spinach, 250ml (9fl oz/1 cup) coconut water and 1 tablespoon ground flaxseed.

Berry greens
Blend together 250ml (9fl oz/1 cup) coconut water or water with a handful each of blueberries, raspberries and strawberries, 1 small banana and a handful of kale. Add a scoop of hemp protein powder if wished.

Hydrating coconut
Juice ½ cucumber with 1 celery stick, 1½ apples and 1 lime. Blend together with 125ml (4fl oz/½ cup) coconut water, 1 tablespoon coconut cream, 1 teaspoon wheatgrass powder or chlorella powder, a pinch of Himalayan salt. Add a small handful of ice if wished.

Omega shake
Put ½ tablespoon chia seeds in a blender and pour over 2 tablespoons water. Leave to soak for 15 minutes. Add 125ml (4fl oz/½ cup) nut milk, 1 tablespoon shelled hemp seeds, ½ teaspoon Manuka honey and 1 frozen, chopped banana. Blend together until creamy.

Tropical pineapple
Blend together 250ml (9fl oz/1 cup) coconut water, 1 small ripe avocado, ¼ pineapple, cut into chunks and 1 tablespoon spirulina or other green food powder. Add 1 teaspoon probiotic powder if wished.

FOOD SENSITIVITIES AND ALLERGIES

As we have already mentioned, the central nervous system (CNS) is connected to the gastro-intestinal tract by what is referred to as the enteric nervous system (ENS), or the gut–brain axis (*see* page 46). What this means is that the health of your gut can directly influence your emotional health. In the same way that anxiety can result in an upset tummy, foods that we are sensitive to can affect brain function.

The digestive system has been described as a "second brain". It produces neurotransmitters (e.g. serotonin), hormones and immune messengers (cytokines) that communicate with the brain. Because of this link any gut-related conditions can have an effect on how we think and feel. For example, cytokines, which are often produced as part of an immune reaction in the gut, can make you feel depressed and reduce levels of serotonin (our feel-good neurotransmitter). In fact, when it is healthy our gut produces much of our serotonin. Therefore, keeping your gut healthy is vital for boosting your mood. One way to do this is by maintaining adequate levels of healthy bacteria (probiotics) in your gut. Probiotics can reduce inflammation and improve the brain receptors' response to neurotransmitters travelling via the gut–brain axis. They are also important in helping the body respond appropriately to the food we eat and reducing the risk of developing food allergies and sensitivities. To boost levels of probiotics, eat natural live yogurt, as well as fermented foods such as miso, nattō, tempeh, kefir and sauerkraut. You may also benefit from taking a supplement.

FOOD ALLERGIES AND THE GUT–BRAIN CONNECTION

The connection between the gut and the brain explains why food allergies and sensitivities have been shown to cause brain-chemistry imbalances and inflammation in the brain affecting mood and behaviour. Food allergies have been linked to a range of

---

BITE-SIZE SOLUTION

Gluten grains are one of the most common food allergens. Gluten is present in wheat, barley, rye and spelt. Oats are often contaminated with gluten and some people find the protein in oats (avenin) also difficult to digest. Good alternatives include rice, quinoa, amaranth, buckwheat, millet, cornflour, maize as well as starchy vegetables like sweet potato and potato.

ALLERGY TRIGGERS

COMMON FOOD ALLERGIES
* Wheat, gluten, dairy, egg, soy, yeast, shellfish, nuts

COMMON FOOD SENSITIVITIES/INTOLERANCES
(Reactions to these food substances do not result in the production of antibodies, as in allergies, but cause similar symptoms.)
* Histamine: found in red wine and beer, fermented cheese, shellfish, fish, tomatoes, chicken, spinach, cured sausage, chocolate, fermented vegetables (sauerkraut) and soy sauce
* Tyramine: found in cheese, beer, wine, bananas, yeast extract, avocados, tinned fish, raspberries, tomatoes, red plums, soy, vinegar and pickles
* Monosodium glutamate (MSG): often added to processed foods, ready meals and takeaways, especially Chinese food
* Solanine: found in the nightshade family – potatoes, peppers, tomatoes and aubergines
* Lactose: found in dairy products

symptoms including hyperactivity, autism, depression, addictive behaviour, irritability, anxiety and aggressive behaviour.

The allergies most likely to influence our mood and behaviour are referred to as delayed food allergies rather than the typical hypersensitivity or acute allergies most people are familiar with, which are known as immediate-acting immunoglobulin E (IgE)-mediated responses.

Delayed, or hidden food allergies, also known as immunoglobulin G (IgG)-mediated responses, can cause systemic low-grade inflammation in the body and this can include inflammation in the brain. Inflammation does not only affect our mood but has been linked to behavioural disorders. Various studies have shown that attention-deficit hyperactivity disorder (ADHD) can improve dramatically through an elimination diet based on IgG food-sensitivity testing.

Allergies and sensitivities can also contribute to food addiction. It has been observed that food-allergic people frequently develop addictions to the foods they are allergic to. Thus the removal of allergic foods can result in the onset of withdrawal symptoms such as headaches, insomnia, irritability, depression, anxiety, mental fogginess, mood swings and fatigue. However, the good news is that these symptoms do not last.

Craving certain foods may be a sign of brain-chemistry imbalances; common allergens such as wheat, dairy, soy and corn can influence brain chemistry creating a temporary feel-good effect. Some of us have enzymes in our digestive tract that break down certain peptides (small chains of amino acids) like gluten into opioids that act like heroin or morphine. This can mean that if these foods are taken out of your diet you may experience withdrawal symptoms. Opioids disrupt brain function by attaching to receptor sites normally meant for neurotransmitters, which explains why foods such as dairy and gluten have been found to play a role in cases of ADHD, autism, or behavioural problems as well as brain fog, anxiety and migraines.

Depression can also be associated with food allergies. It is a common symptom of untreated coeliac disease – an autoimmune condition triggered by gluten found in wheat, barley and rye. Addictions – for example, to alcohol – have also been linked to depression. This is often due to abnormally low levels of serotonin and/or noradrenalin in the brain.

DO YOU SUFFER FROM A FOOD ALLERGY OR SENSITIVITY?

Tick on the list below any symptoms that you experience regularly:

- [ ] seasonal allergies, hayfever
- [ ] asthma or eczema
- [ ] daily mood swings
- [ ] lethargy or apathy, particularly after eating
- [ ] feeling better if you don't eat certain foods
- [ ] unexplained grogginess/fatigue
- [ ] headaches or migraines
- [ ] low mood
- [ ] inflammatory bowel conditions such as colitis or Crohn's disease
- [ ] poor concentration
- [ ] muscle aches and pains
- [ ] dark circles under your eyes
- [ ] fluid retention and weight gain after eating certain foods
- [ ] food cravings, such as for bread or cheese
- [ ] irritable bowel syndrome/constipation/mild diarrhoea

If you've ticked more than two or three of the above symptoms you may be suffering from a food allergy.

FOOD ALLERGY AND SENSITIVITY TESTING

If you suspect you have an allergy or sensitivity then consider taking a blood test with a qualified practitioner. IgG blood tests can help you identify any foods you are currently eating that cause a delayed reaction and assess how severe that response is. You may suspect you are reacting to gluten; if so, you should also test for coeliac disease. Being gluten-sensitive isn't black and white. There are degrees of sensitivity. And not all sensitivity to wheat is, strictly speaking, a gluten sensitivity. It has been discovered that wheat comprises more than 100 different components that can cause a reaction. New tests are now available that will look for these other components in addition to gluten.

If you do react to gluten you may also be sensitive to other foods. This is because proteins in different foods can cross react. In cross-reactivity, the body mistakes another food for gluten and reacts in the same way. Cross-reactivity is common between gluten and dairy, as the structure of dairy closely resembles that of gluten. It is estimated that 50% of people who are sensitive to gluten are also sensitive to dairy. Gluten sensitivity is often hereditary – 98% of people with coeliac disease have a genetic predisposition. If there is a history of gluten sensitivity in your family, you may wish to consider a separate DNA test to look for genetic markers.

If you don't want to undertake tests for food allergies, another approach is to exclude suspected foods from your diet for two weeks, one food at a time, then reintroduce them in a controlled way – recording your symptoms under the guidance of a nutritionist.

If there are foods to which you are reacting, you need to stop eating them to reduce damage and inflammation in the gut. Foods that evoke an immediate IgE-type reaction may need to be avoided for life. If you are diagnosed with coeliac disease you need to avoid gluten for life. IgG food reactions can be short-lived if you take steps to restore gut health and improve digestion, so you may only need to avoid these foods for 3 to 6 months. After you reintroduce such foods, reduce the risk of the sensitivity recurring by eating them only every four or five days to give your gut time to recover.

GOOD-MOOD SUMMARY

If you suspect you have a food allergy/sensitivity:

* start a food diary and look at the common foods you eat and/or crave
* get yourself tested with the support of a nutritionist or qualified healthcare practitioner
* eliminate allergens from your diet and take steps to improve digestion and gut health
* consider gut healing supplements with the advice of a qualified nutritionist
* try to avoid medications (e.g. pain killers, antibiotics) that can damage the digestive tract
* minimize your intake of alcohol and caffeine

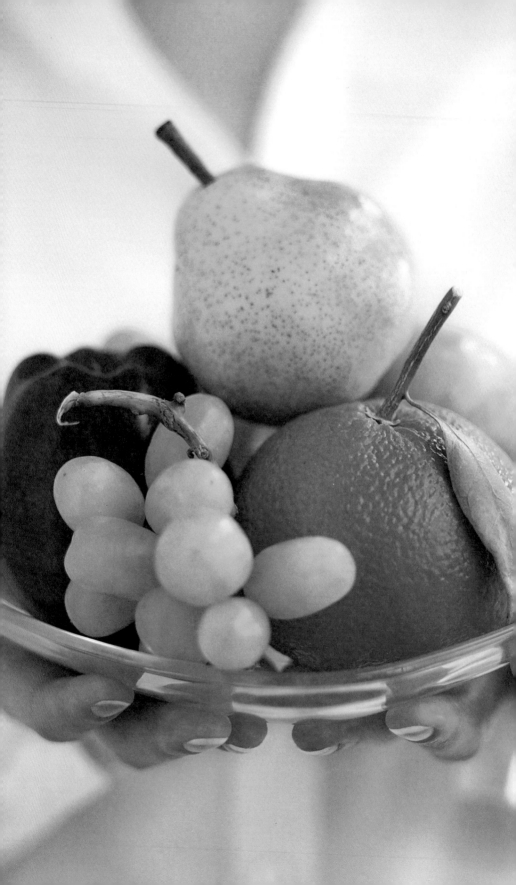

MOOD'S MANY GUISES

The direct link between mood disorders and physical health conditions is becoming increasingly well understood and recognized. By getting to grips with the nutritional factor – or, more often, combination of factors – at the root of our low moods, we are able to see practical, realistic and sustainable ways to address conditions that interfere with our quality of life.

Conditions that affect your mood, mind and energy come in many forms and even more degrees of seriousness. You may feel persistently low; you may find that you are more irritable or turning to food for a boost; you may suffer from premenstrual syndrome or seasonal affective disorder; you may have difficulty sleeping or find your brain power is not what it used to be. One thing all these problems have in common is that they can be closely linked to your diet. In the following pages, we examine in detail a number of mood-related conditions, such as fatigue and depression, and explore how to overcome them using nutritional methods.

HOW TO USE THIS CHAPTER

The information in this chapter is aimed at helping you identify and treat the underlying causes of your current symptoms. However, the advice and guidelines do not replace medical care and it is important you also seek the support of a healthcare practitioner if symptoms appear particularly severe or show little sign of improvement. If you are currently receiving medical care then please check with your healthcare practitioner before implementing major changes to your diet and/or taking nutritional or herbal supplements.

Everyone is unique and therefore you need to adopt a personalized approach to improving your mood, energy and well-being. The checklists at the beginning of each section will help you identify which systems in your body are out of balance – whether it be, for example, your hormones or your gut health or your immune system, or a combination of more than one system.

Everyone who feels their mood, mind or energy could do with a boost will benefit from the basic principles of the diet and lifestyle changes mentioned in this book. However, depending on your answers to the following sections, you may need to add a few extra self-care steps to adapt the programme to your individual needs. In some cases you will need to seek support from a nutritionist who can undertake diagnostic testing as well as advising more specifically on diet and supplements.

The previous chapter outlined the underlying principles of good nutrition, particularly in relation to mood. This chapter is designed to bring together the dietary guidelines that are particularly helpful in treating each mood disorder. You could simply read the section on the condition that interests you. However, for more detail, refer back to sections in Chapter 1, "The Physiology of Melancholy", or forward to Chapter 3, "Feel-Good Food", for advice on how to put those nutritional principles into practice.

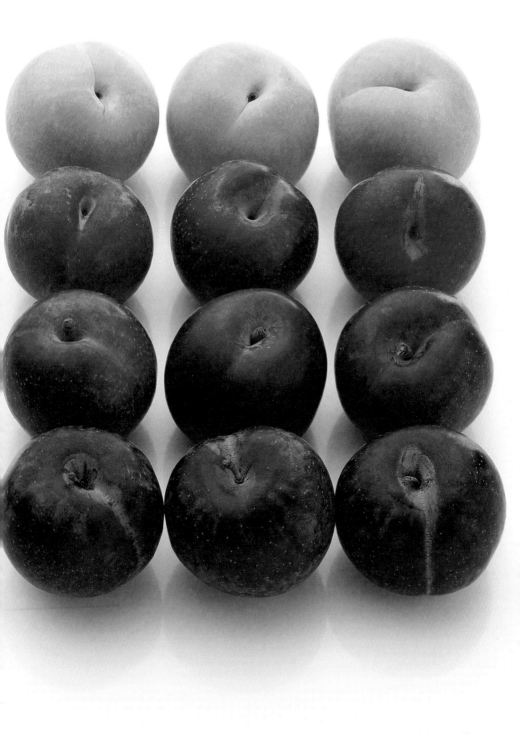

LOW ENERGY

The average diet is high in so-called "empty" calories – or in other words, it is energy-rich and nutrient-poor. Yet without an optimal intake of the nutrients needed to convert calories into usable energy you are likely to end up feeling constantly exhausted, on edge and irritable. By consuming whole, fresh, unprocessed food and drinks, and avoiding substances that drain your energy, you really can tackle ongoing tiredness.

There are certain key nutrients that are important for energy production (*see* table, opposite) and blood-sugar balance (*see* pages 16–25). Low levels of these can contribute to a range of signs and symptoms. On the list below, tick any of the symptoms that are familiar and persistent for you. This will help you determine whether you are low in certain key energy-supporting nutrients.

- ☐ feel tired often
- ☐ regularly get constipated
- ☐ experience muscle twitching and leg/hand cramps
- ☐ experience premenstrual symptoms
- ☐ get anxious or find it hard to unwind
- ☐ experience sleep problems and/or insomnia
- ☐ feel irritable or depressed often
- ☐ experience cravings
- ☐ feel stressed a lot of the time
- ☐ regularly consume coffee, tea, cigarettes or alcohol
- ☐ difficulty concentrating
- ☐ mental fogginess
- ☐ regularly get infections

If you ticked more than three of these, it is likely you will experience benefit from boosting your intake of key energy-supporting nutrients.

BITE-SIZE SOLUTION

To get each day off to a good start, boost your energy levels by having a protein-based breakfast such as an omelette with vegetables. This will prevent your blood sugar – and your energy and mood – from plummeting mid-morning, leaving you reaching for a pick-me-up, such as a coffee or sugary pastry.

KEY ENERGY NUTRIENTS

The following list shows the food sources of energy-boosting nutrients:

NUTRIENT	RICH FOOD SOURCES
Vitamin B1	Beef kidney and liver, brewer's yeast, brown rice, chickpeas, kidney beans, pork, rice bran, salmon, soya beans, sunflower seeds, wheatgerm, whole-grain wheat and rye
Vitamin B2	Almonds, brewer's yeast, cheese, chicken, mushrooms, wheatgerm
Vitamin B3	Beef liver, brewer's yeast, chicken, eggs, fish, sunflower seeds, turkey
Vitamin B5	Blue cheese, brewer's yeast, corn, eggs, lentils, liver, lobster, meats, peanuts, peas, soya beans, sunflower seeds, wheatgerm, whole-grain products
Vitamin B6	Avocados, bananas, bran, brewer's yeast, carrots, hazelnuts, lentils, rice, salmon, shrimps, soya beans, sunflower seeds, tuna, walnuts, wheatgerm, whole-grain flour
Vitamin C	Blackcurrants, broccoli, Brussels sprouts, cabbage, grapefruit, green peppers, guava, kale, lemons, oranges, papaya, potatoes, spinach, strawberries, tomatoes, watercress
Chromium	Beef, brewer's yeast, chicken, eggs, fish, fruit, milk products, potatoes, whole grains
Coenzyme Q10	All foods, particularly beef, mackerel, sardines, soya oil, spinach
Magnesium	Almonds, fish, green leafy vegetables, kelp, molasses, nuts, soya beans, sunflower seeds, wheatgerm
Zinc	Egg yolk, fish, all meat, milk, molasses, oysters, sesame seeds, soya beans, sunflower seeds, turkey, wheatgerm, whole grains

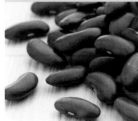
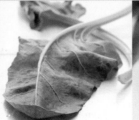
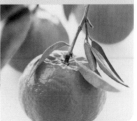

ACTIVE INGREDIENT: B VITAMINS

Inside each cell in your body are minute energy factories called mitochondria. How much energy you feel you have and, to a large degree, the quality of your moods depends on the production of energy inside every single one of these microscopic powerhouses. For energy to be created, a combustion process takes place. To fuel this process, the mitochondria require a constant supply of glucose, oxygen and nutrients. Among the key nutrient players are vitamins B1, B3, B5, B6 and biotin (another B vitamin). B vitamins are also needed to help maintain healthy nerves and to produce the important neurotransmitters (brain messenger molecules) that help maintain mood and control appetite.

When we are under stress, we tend to turn to refined foods (from which much of the B-vitamin content has been removed). So, although our demand for B vitamins is higher at these times, our intake of them may actually be lower than normal. You should get into the habit of including plenty of foods that are rich in B vitamins in your diet, so that you naturally persist with them during crunch times. Particularly good sources of B vitamins include: brewer's yeast, brown rice and other whole grains, sunflower seeds, wheatgerm, nuts, eggs, fish, lean meat and poultry (*see* also the table on page 65).

However, increasing your B-vitamin supplies is only part of the story: you also need to minimize your intake of those tempting, but B-vitamin depleted refined foods. *For example, refined white flour contains less than a quarter of the level of vitamin B1 and a fifth of the B3 found in its whole-grain counterpart.* Try also to steer clear of substances that hamper the absorption and use of B vitamins in the body. Alcohol, caffeine and some medical drugs, including the contraceptive pill, are all culprits.

In addition to eating a diet rich in fresh, whole foods and avoiding refined foods, taking a B-complex vitamin supplement (or a multivitamin that is high in B vitamins) can help ensure that you are getting enough of these important nutrients. Do remember, though, that supplements are not a substitute for eating well, cutting out stimulants and getting enough sleep. The following recipes from Chapter 3 are particularly rich in B vitamins:

BREAKFASTS: Berry Brain Smoothie (page 117); Nut and Seed Muesli (page 120)
LIGHT MEAL: Baby Spinach, Avocado and Goat's Cheese Salad (page 121)
MAIN MEALS: Frittata (page 142); Lentils with Spinach (page 154)
DESSERT: Walnut Oat Crumble (page 170)

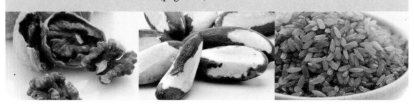

While optimizing your intake of certain nutrients is likely to be beneficial for everyone, a lack of these nutrients may not be the sole reason for your ongoing fatigue. For example, optimizing digestion and absorption of nutrients and eliminating toxins are equally important for supporting energy levels. Similarly, ensuring your blood-sugar levels are balanced, identifying and excluding food allergens and tackling chronic stress can make all the difference.

Other culprits may include hormonal, thyroid and adrenal imbalances as well as disturbances in circadian rhythm leading to poor sleep (*see* pages 81–5).

EATING FOR ENERGY

The link between your diet and how energetic you feel is easy to see – after all, we know that if we drank a strong coffee and ate a bar of chocolate we would be buzzing, for a while at least. On a cellular level, we are, with our diets, literally fuelling all our cells to produce energy through a carefully controlled chemical reaction. The type of fuel we use correlates to our performance, much like that of a car. In fact, many of us may be more careful about fuelling and servicing our cars than we are our own bodies!

To produce energy, each cell needs a supply of fuel in the form of glucose, derived from carbohydrates and, to a lesser extent, fats in our diet. However, the process of

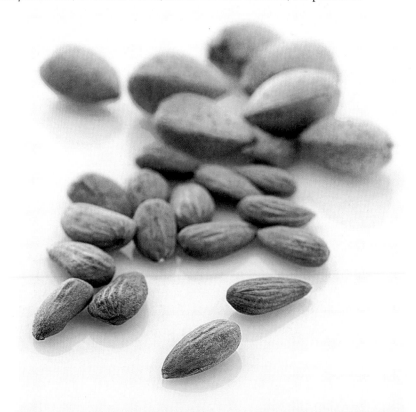

converting the fuel into energy requires a range of micro-nutrients. Ensuring you take in the full range is best achieved by basing your diet around fresh, unprocessed organic foods. See the table on page 65 for a list of foods that are rich in energy-boosting nutrients, and pages 181–3 for more on a nutrient-rich diet. If you have ticked many of the symptoms on page 64, you may also need to consider taking a quality multivitamin and mineral supplement.

Avoiding foods that sap your energy is just as important as eating energy-rich foods. The energy drainers include stimulants such as caffeine, alcohol and sugar – these play havoc with our blood-sugar levels (for more on the mechanism controlling blood-sugar levels, *see* pages 16–25).

COFFEE: FRIEND OR FOE?

If you are experiencing low energy and/or poor sleep, you should eliminate coffee and caffeine from your diet – at least to begin with. Caffeine is a drug that may initially boost our energy but ultimately will deplete our reserves, leading to an energy crash and potentially to cravings. The detrimental effects of excessive caffeine intake are well documented; they include addiction, gastric upset and disrupted sleep. Caffeine has a powerful (and negative) effect on blood-sugar balance and in turn affects energy levels. Often people get trapped in a vicious cycle of using coffee to perk up energy levels in an effort to compensate for a night's sleep that has been disrupted by too much caffeine the day before.

However, there is research to suggest that in some respects regular coffee drinking may benefit health. It has been shown to improve athletic endurance, mood and cognition. It may also reduce the risk of Alzheimer's disease. Coffee contains a range of antioxidants including polyphenols (particularly chlorogenic acid), which may be responsible for some of its health benefits. However, if you are using it to keep up energy levels – or you feel jittery or irritable without it – it is likely you are addicted to caffeine and therefore you should eliminate it from your diet. Decaffeinated (organic) varieties would be a better option.

Removing caffeine from your diet can lead initially to withdrawal symptoms such as headaches and can leave you feeling more tired for the first few days. However, over the longer term you should find your energy levels begin to improve. To reduce the impact of withdrawal symptoms, you might start removing it at the weekend to allow you to catch up on sleep. In addition, make sure you drink plenty of water through the day and gradually cut down your intake rather than immediately cutting it out. Some people find that taking a vitamin C supplement (1000mg) daily can be helpful.

ENERGY-BOOSTING RECIPES

BREAKFAST: Scrambled Eggs on Rye with Leeks and Mushrooms (page 114)
LIGHT MEALS: Mediterranean Chicken Salad (page 122); Mixed Bean and Goat's
Cheese Salad with Lemon Oil Dressing (page 130); Chicken Liver and Antipasto
Salad (page 131); Mackerel Pâté (page 126)
MAIN MEALS: Sweet Roast Lamb (page 150); Shiitake Chicken (page 153); Turmeric
and Tamarind Glazed Salmon (page 144)
DESSERTS: Lemon Coconut Bars (page 171); Maca Ice Cream (page 171)

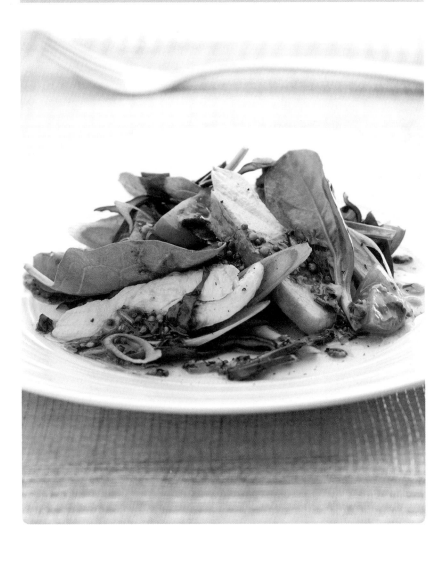

PREMENSTRUAL SYNDROME (PMS)

Many women suffer the effects of premenstrual syndrome (PMS) in varying degrees every month. These may include symptoms such as irritability or cravings through to serious mood swings and emotional unpredictability. PMS is a disorder that generally manifests itself in the two weeks leading up to menstruation. It can affect a woman at any stage of her reproductive life and can produce a wide range of physical and emotional changes.

Look at the list below and tick any of those that apply to you:
- [ ] bloating, change in bowel movements
- [ ] weight gain
- [ ] breast tenderness
- [ ] headache/migraine
- [ ] pelvic discomfort and pain
- [ ] increase in appetite and/or cravings
- [ ] irritability
- [ ] anxiety
- [ ] mood swings
- [ ] loss of concentration
- [ ] depression
- [ ] brain fog
- [ ] crying spells/tearfulness
- [ ] clumsiness

If you experience any of the above symptoms in the 10 days or so before your period, which ease after the start of menstruation, then it is likely that you are affected by PMS.

BITE-SIZE SOLUTION

If you find water retention and bloating a problem, just before your period try to keep your diet low in salt and increase your consumption of potassium (good sources include baked potato, beans and pulses) and magnesium (found in leafy green vegetables, nuts and seeds). Drink plenty of water and coconut water and reduce your intake of foods with a high salt content (processed foods, condiments, cheese, snack foods).

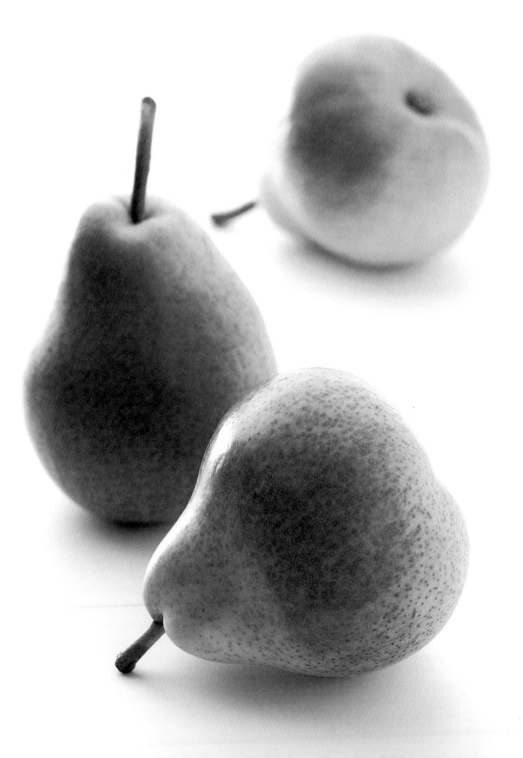

ACTIVE INGREDIENT: PHYTO-OESTROGENS

The delicate balance between the oestrogen and progesterone in your body can be disturbed by exposure to many man-made chemicals, such as pharmaceuticals (for example, drugs), agrochemicals (including pesticides and fertilizers) and petrochemicals (such as plastics). These chemicals contain toxic xeno-oestrogens ("xeno" means external), which can act similarly to strong oestrogens in the body, worsening PMS symptoms, as well as other female reproductive disorders such as endometriosis and infertility.

Phyto-oestrogens are substances similar in structure to oestrogens that occur naturally in plants. They have a balancing effect on our hormones when they are either too low or too high. This makes them useful for PMS and menopausal symptoms. If our oestrogen levels are low phyto-oestrogens lock onto oestrogen receptors in cells and boost levels. However, when our oestrogen levels are too high these same phyto-oestrogens lock onto the oestrogen receptors and give a weak oestrogenic effect that blocks out the effects of xeno-oestrogens, thereby reducing our overall oestrogen levels.

While phyto-oestrogens are present in many fruits, vegetables and grains, one of the most concentrated sources is soya. Soya is naturally rich in phyto-oestrogenic compounds called isoflavones. Traditionally soya is eaten in the form of fermented whole foods, such as miso, tempeh and nattō. This fermentation converts the phyto-oestrogenic isoflavones into their absorbable and active form, making them much more effective. Including foods naturally rich in phyto-oestrogens daily may therefore be helpful in easing the symptoms of PMS. Other foods rich in phyto-oestrogens include flaxseed, hummus, garlic, alfalfa, sunflower seeds, almonds, licorice, beans, sesame seeds and herbs such as sage, parsley and basil.

The following recipes are rich in phyto-oestrogens:

BREAKFAST: Nut and Seed Muesli (page 120)

LIGHT MEALS: Hummus, Avocado and Alfalfa baked-potato topping (page 124); Mixed Bean and Goat's Cheese Salad (page 130); Supergreens Salad (page 161)

MAIN MEALS: Lentils with Spinach (page 154); Spiced Bean Stew (page 157)

DESSERT: Walnut Oat Crumble (page 170)

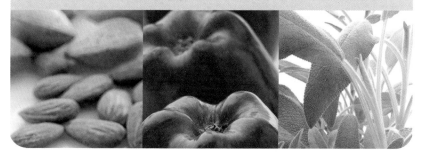

There are a number of factors that are thought to play a role in the symptoms of PMS including hormonal and biological imbalances, nutritional insufficiencies as well as psychological factors.

HORMONAL BALANCE

One of the key causes of PMS symptoms is an imbalance between the hormones oestrogen and progesterone. If you take the contraceptive pill, which contains progestin (a synthetic substance whose effect is similar to progesterone), you may have too much progesterone in your body. Other cases of progesterone excess, especially those associated with depression, can be attributed to falling oestrogen levels just before the start of the period.

However, it is more commonly an excess of oestrogen that brings about PMS symptoms. There are a number of reasons why this may occur: for example, your ovaries may not be secreting enough progesterone, your liver and gut may not be eliminating oestrogen efficiently enough, or you may be taking oestrogen in from external sources such as medications or environmental pollutants.

The liver plays a vital role in recycling and breaking down hormones, including oestrogen, so supporting the liver detoxification pathways (*see* pages 48–51) can make a significant difference in improving oestrogen–progesterone balance. B-vitamin insufficiencies, especially of vitamin B6, as well as low levels of magnesium, can decrease the liver's ability to detoxify oestrogen. By supplementing with these nutrients dramatic improvements in symptoms can be made.

BLOOD-SUGAR IMBALANCES

There is also research linking PMS to low blood sugar. We have already discussed how dips in blood sugar can trigger symptoms such as irritability, anxiety, cravings for sweet foods and low mood. Therefore, it is crucial to follow the guidelines to help you balance blood-sugar levels (*see* pages 16–25).

THE MOOD–PMS LINK

One reason why low mood is often linked to PMS is that high levels of oestrogen can suppress the action of dopamine, our "motivating" neurotransmitter. To compensate for this effect eat foods rich in vitamin B6, vitamin C and magnesium, as well as the amino acid tyrosine, which are all required for production of dopamine.

On the other hand, women who are low in oestrogen are often low in serotonin, a neurotransmitter involved in regulating mood, appetite and sleep patterns. This is because oestrogen prevents serotonin from breaking down and leaving the body, thereby prolonging its positive effect on your mood. This problem can be particularly marked just before menstruation, when oestrogen levels are generally at their lowest. See the advice on boosting serotonin levels on page 96.

STRESS AND PROLACTIN

Some women with PMS have abnormally high levels of a hormone called prolactin. This is often due to high stress since stress depletes dopamine, which in turn leads to an increase in levels of prolactin. High prolactin can cause an imbalance between oestrogen and progesterone and symptoms such as breast tenderness and swelling, anxiety and irritability. Prolactin levels can be raised for other reasons too such as low levels of key nutrients including B vitamins and magnesium as well as an underactive thyroid.

INFLAMMATION

Some of the symptoms of PMS, such as cramps, backache, breast tenderness and headaches, indicate the presence of inflammation. Including anti-inflammatory nutrients such as essential fatty acids in your diet (*see* pages 40–43) can be helpful.

NUTRITIONAL SUPPORT

While there is a range of factors that can contribute to the symptoms of PMS, you should in any case include foods in your diet that are rich in key nutrients shown to support hormonal balance. These include B vitamins especially B3 and B6, vitamin C, magnesium, zinc and chromium. You may also wish to include a supplement containing these nutrients. Other supportive nutrients shown to alleviate PMS symptoms include vitamin E, omega 3 fats and starflower oil (borage oil), which contains gamma linolenic acid (GLA), an essential omega 6 fat.

Include herbs to support digestion, liver function and adrenals too. These include fennel, dandelion, milk thistle, hops and ginseng.

Agnus castus is a herb popularly used for many PMS symptoms. It acts on the pituitary gland aiding the secretion of progesterone and therefore helps to balance high oestrogen levels. It also inhibits the secretion of prolactin.

RECIPES TO COMBAT PMS

BREAKFASTS: Buckwheat Crêpes (page 117); Apple Porridge (page 116); Berry Brain Smoothie (page 117)

LIGHT MEALS: Baby Spinach, Avocado and Goat's Cheese Salad (page 121); Puy Lentil Salad (page 133); Fish Soup Provençale (page 138); Bean and Courgette Soup with Pesto (page 139); Quinoa Tabouleh (page 162)

MAIN MEALS: Trout with Sunflower Seeds (page 147); Salmon Rolls (page 147); Spiced Bean Stew (page 157)

DESSERTS: Maca Ice Cream (page 171); Walnut Oat Crumble (page 170)

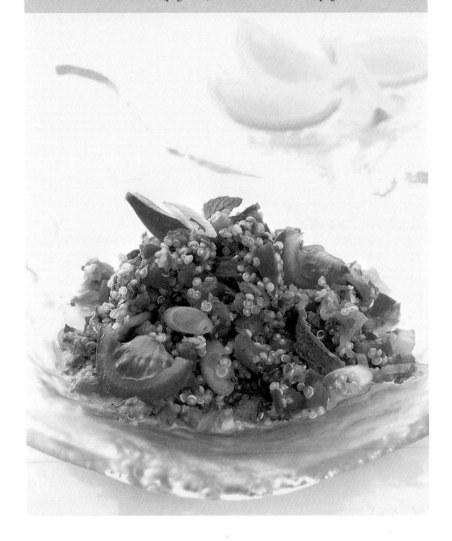

SEASONAL AFFECTIVE DISORDER (SAD)

Seasonal affective disorder (SAD) is a condition that is characterized by low mood brought on by reduced exposure to sunlight. Generally, this seasonal sadness will begin in the autumn or winter, and disappear in the spring. The condition is common, with estimates of one in twenty people being affected to some degree. SAD sufferers often experience extreme tiredness and sleep more than usual. They may also experience an increase in appetite and weight during the winter months.

As SAD is essentially caused by lack of sunlight, it is important to get as much natural daylight as possible. Your levels of vitamin D are also important. It is estimated that around 70–80% of the UK and US population are deficient in vitamin D.

Look at the list below and tick any symptoms you experience over the autumn and winter months:

- [ ] increased sleep
- [ ] feeling unrefreshed after sleep
- [ ] craving starchy and sweet foods
- [ ] overeating
- [ ] sore or weak muscles
- [ ] mental fog
- [ ] weight gain
- [ ] feelings of hopelessness
- [ ] irritability
- [ ] anxiety
- [ ] inability to concentrate
- [ ] lethargy, lack of motivation

If you ticked five or more symptoms, you may suffer from SAD.

THE IMPORTANCE OF VITAMIN D

While the role of vitamin D in supporting bone health has long been recognized, recent research has also shown its importance in reducing the risk of cardiovascular disease, certain cancers and diabetes. It is known to improve immune function and

THE IMPORTANCE OF LIGHT

The control centre in our brain that determines our moods and daily rhythms is governed in part by the amount of light that enters our eyes. When light hits certain parts of the retina, it affects the release of the hormone melatonin. During the night, or in darkness, melatonin production increases, making us sleepy. When day breaks and our eyes are exposed to natural light, melatonin production stops.

During the dark winter days, therefore, the control mechanism for melatonin release changes. It appears that SAD sufferers are especially sensitive to this change.

Light- or phototherapy, is a treatment for SAD involving daily exposure to high-intensity, broad-spectrum artificial light from a light box, in order to suppress the production of melatonin. Phototherapy may also help to increase levels of the mood-boosting neurotransmitter serotonin. It may therefore be worth considering purchasing a light box for use at home or work. These devices, which give off light with the specific characteristics of the sun's rays, can often help to combat the symptoms of SAD.

several studies reveal its role in combating depression, low mood and SAD. A low level of vitamin D is also linked with an increased risk of cognitive decline in the over-65s.

Your body makes most of its own vitamin D when your skin is exposed to sunshine, which means that levels can fall dramatically during the autumn and winter months. There are also a few foods that are rich in vitamin D, including mackerel and herring, and porcini or shiitake mushrooms.

If you are suffering from symptoms related to SAD, low mood or reduced cognitive function, you should get your vitamin D level tested by a qualified nutritionist. If your levels are low (below 60–70nmol/ml), you should get more sun, eat 3–4 servings of oily fish a week and take a supplement.

Even on a dull day, you will still benefit from spending time outside. The amount of natural light available outdoors is higher than levels found in most indoor settings. Try brisk walking, jogging or cycling to get a double mood-boost – from exercise as well as daylight.

COMBATING FOOD CRAVINGS

Sufferers of SAD often have reduced levels of serotonin during the winter months. Serotonin plays an important role in regulating appetite – when we are low in serotonin, we often feel more hungry. As many carbohydrate foods are rich in tryptophan, the precursor to serotonin, this may explain why those experiencing SAD tend to

SUPPLEMENTARY SUPPORT

Many SAD sufferers find that taking a preparation based on the herb hypericum (St John's wort) helps relieve their symptoms. Hypericum has been shown in studies to boost mood – through, it is believed, optimizing serotonin function. Other useful supportive supplements include liquid iodine, vitamin D, essential fatty acids and 5HTP. Note that St John's wort commonly interacts with medications so please seek support from your healthcare practitioner before taking this herb.

reach for starchy foods like bread, pasta and pastries. The trouble is that these foods can cause imbalances in blood-sugar levels, which can trigger further increases in appetite and cravings. There are, however, healthy sources of tryptophan. Eating these foods regularly may help the body produce more serotonin and boost mood without disrupting blood-sugar levels. See the box on page 96 for details on foods to include.

Another neurotransmitter, dopamine, may also play a role in SAD. Some studies have indicated that dopamine levels increase when bright light hits the back of the eye. As dopamine is thought to improve alertness, concentration and motivation, reduced levels in darker months could explain in part some of the symptoms of SAD, such as lethargy and low mood. Increasing your intake of foods rich in the amino acids tyrosine and phenylalanine, which the body can convert into dopamine, may help. Good food sources include lean meat, dairy products, fish and eggs.

If you suffer with food cravings try the following:

* Balance blood sugar (*see* pages 16–25). Swings in blood sugar are one of the major causes of cravings so keep blood sugar stable. Eliminate sugars, fizzy drinks, fruit juice, artificial sweeteners and refined carbohydrates. Combine good protein foods with healthy fats (*see* pages 38–43) and slow-releasing carbohydrates.
* Eat a protein breakfast. Including protein at breakfast helps reduce cravings and control appetite. Try a protein shake, nuts and seeds, eggs and fish.
* Include snacks during the day. Eat a couple of healthy protein-rich snacks during the day and do not allow yourself to become too hungry.
* Avoid eating within three hours of bedtime. This can actually increase insulin levels and may increase cravings as well as disturb blood sugar and sleep patterns.
* Get sufficient vitamin D – not only is this important for boosting mood, low levels of vitamin D may also impair your appetite control.
* Take natural supplements for cravings. Consider a supplement to help balance blood sugar that includes chromium. L-glutamine powder can also be very effective.

* Include soluble fibre – this helps you feel fuller for longer and aids blood-sugar control. Eat foods such as beans, pulses, oats, nuts, seeds, vegetables and fruit such as apples and pears.

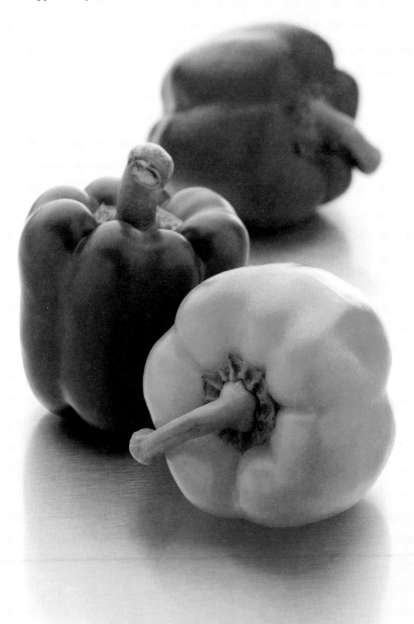

RECIPES TO EASE SAD

BREAKFASTS: Apple Porridge (page 116); Nut and Seed Muesli (page 120); Poached Eggs with Asparagus (page 118)

LIGHT MEALS: Chicken and Mushroom Pâté (page 128); Chicken Liver and Antipasto Salad (page 131); Mackerel Pâté (page 126)

MAIN MEALS: Herbed Rice Salad with Salmon (page 126); Frittata (page 142); Stuffed Vegetables (page 142); Sweet Roast Lamb (page 150); Trout with Sunflower Seeds (page 147)

DESSERT: Chocolate Banana Mousse (page 170)

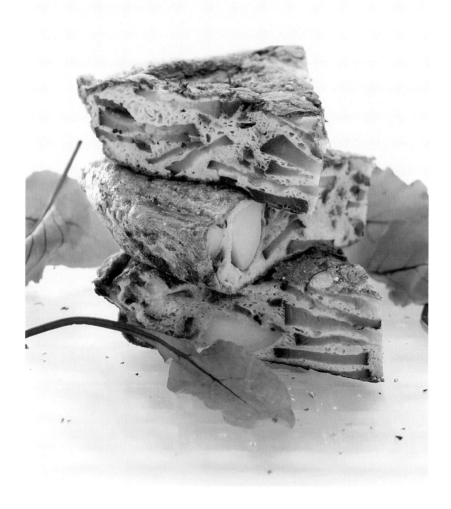

TROUBLE SLEEPING

Modern living is not generally a recipe for good sleep, or enough of it. Faced with the stresses of our 24/7 culture, many of us go to bed later than we should, and when we do finally turn in we may find it difficult to drop off to sleep or repeatedly wake up during the night. Missing out on quality sleep not only makes us feel low the next day but can impact on our overall state of health in the longer term.

On the list below, tick the symptoms that commonly apply to you:
- difficulty getting to sleep
- waking up in the night
- waking early and not getting back to sleep
- feeling unrefreshed after a night's sleep
- putting off going to bed, even when tired
- energy slumps/dozing during the day
- falling asleep early in the evening but not sleeping well at night
- daytime drowsiness
- impatience and/or irritability
- difficulty remembering or retaining information
- making frequent errors or mistakes
- low mood regularly
- feeling you could doze off when sitting, reading or watching television

If you ticked four or more symptoms, you could probably benefit from altering your diet and lifestyle in order to improve the quality and amount of sleep you are getting. An ongoing sleeplessness problem can affect productivity and relationships. Without adequate sleep, the body quickly shows clear signs of stress. Sleep deprivation makes us tired, moody and irritable and, in the long term, even depressed. Sleep-deprived individuals have also been found to have a reduction in the immune cells needed to resist invaders, reducing their ability to fight off illness and infection.

Sleep is made up of a series of regular sleep cycles of varying lengths and depths. In the average healthy person, the whole sleep cycle, including stage four (the deepest kind of sleep), lasts roughly 90 minutes. The first two complete sleep cycles are thought to contain mostly stage three and four sleep, during which the body releases growth hormone, which stimulates regeneration and repair of cells, burns fat, stimulates metabolism and supports immune function. REM (dream sleep) occurs mainly in

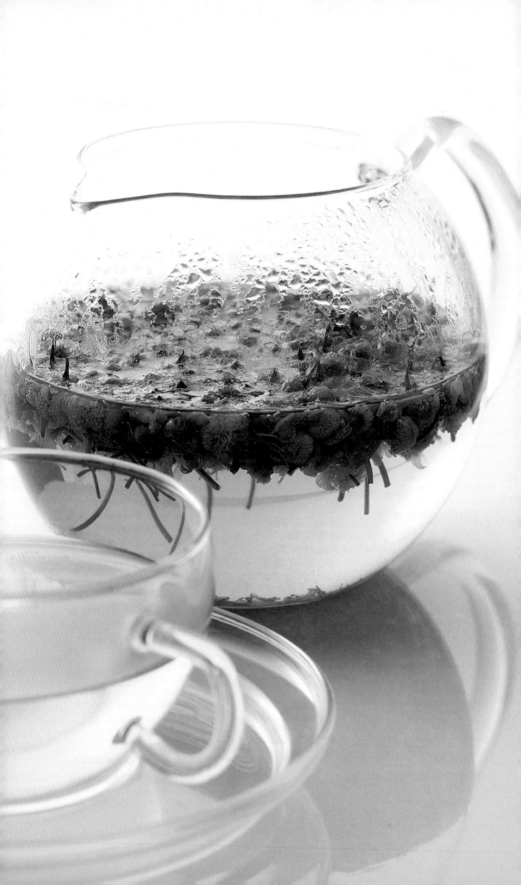

GOOD SLEEP HABITS

As well as considering nutritional strategies, you should think about your sleep regime and environment (referred to by experts as "sleep hygiene") and make changes, if necessary. Here are some top tips:

- Make sure your bedroom is quiet, dark and at a comfortable temperature.
- Avoid eating a large meal during the three hours before you go to bed.
- Do not exercise within three hours of going to bed.
- Keep your bedroom for sleeping – remove all electrical equipment including televisions and mobile phones.
- Take a warm bath before bed, perhaps adding a calming aromatherapy oil such as lavender to the water.
- Avoid coffee or alcohol in the afternoon or evening.
- Wear loose comfortable clothing in bed.
- Eat regularly through the day to balance blood sugar.

the second half of the sleep period; and lighter sleep (stages one and two) comes only at the end of the night. If you are deprived of sleep for a while, at the earliest opportunity your body will try to make up this deficit by quickly going to stage four and REM sleep in each cycle. However, if we do not go through all these stages of sleep in their correct proportions we will not feel refreshed or rejuvenated.

SEEKING HELP

If you are suffering from insomnia you may wish to seek support of a healthcare practitioner or nutritionist. Insomnia can be a symptom of chronic anxiety, depression or stress rather than the cause, and will often improve if you are able to address the underlying problem. Diagnostic tests can be undertaken to measure levels of cortisol and adrenalin, which are often elevated in people suffering from chronic insomnia. High levels of these hormones before bedtime will interfere with your production of the sleep-regulating hormone melatonin as well as the calming neurotransmitter GABA. By looking at your sleep-wake cycle you can take appropriate supplements to rebalance your circadian rhythm.

FALSE FRIENDS

When our sleep quality is impaired, it can be tempting to resort to stimulants such as coffee to keep us alert during the day then turn to alcohol in the evening to help us relax. Alcohol promotes GABA and switches off adrenalin, but it will only do this for a couple of hours. Unfortunately, alcohol also disturbs blood-sugar levels, which can lead to night-time waking. Going to sleep under the influence of alcohol disrupts your sleep cycle and over the long term will actually deplete GABA. Caffeine will raise adrenalin and disturb blood-sugar levels further upsetting your sleep.

When sleep problems become severe, sleeping pills may seem to offer an obvious solution, but beware of their highly addictive nature and their tendency to cause day-time drowsiness and poor mental function.

NUTRIENTS FOR SLEEP

The amino acid tryptophan, which is converted to 5-hydroxytryptophan (5HTP) and then to serotonin, which boosts our mood, is also the raw material for melatonin – the hormone to help you sleep. Therefore, eating foods rich in tryptophan – such as bananas, chicken, figs, milk, oats, seaweed, sunflower seeds, tuna, eggs, nuts, turkey and yogurt – may help in inducing sleep. You will also need to boost your intake of certain vitamins and minerals required to convert tryptophan into melatonin, particularly folic acid, vitamins B6 and C and zinc.

The following snacks and light meals are rich in tryptophan and should therefore help you sleep:

- oatcakes with tuna or a slice of chicken/turkey
- oatcakes with tahini, hummus, nut butter or cottage cheese
- a small pot of natural yogurt with sunflower seeds and a banana
- banana protein shake (with milk or soya milk)
- handful of sunflower seeds or almonds

Other beneficial nutrients include magnesium and calcium, which are calming and aid muscle relaxation. Magnesium has been reported to help restless legs as well as insomnia. Good sources of calcium include milk, green vegetables and nuts. Magnesium is found in seeds, nuts, green vegetables and seafood (*see also* the table on page 183). Taking a magnesium supplement in the evening may also help. While B vitamins are important for tackling ongoing stress, you should take them earlier in the day as they can be energizing and therefore may interfere with your sleep.

There are also certain herbs that have been shown to aid sleep. One of the best known is valerian, which helps promote GABA. It is best taken in the evening for this reason, but avoid taking it in conjunction with alcohol or sleeping pills. Other beneficial herbs include chamomile, passion flower, hops and lemon balm.

RECIPES FOR IMPROVED SLEEP

You are more likely to sleep well if you eat a lighter meal in the early evening. Include foods that contain tryptophan too. Here are some ideas:

BREAKFASTS: Apple Porridge (page 116); Yogurt Fruit Bowl (page 114)

LIGHT MEALS: Baby Spinach, Avocado and Goat's Cheese Salad (page 121); Root Vegetable Soup (page 134)

MAIN MEALS: Stuffed Vegetables (page 142); Mediterranean Chicken Salad (page 136)

DESSERTS: Chocolate Banana Mousse (page 170); Walnut Oat Crumble (page 170)

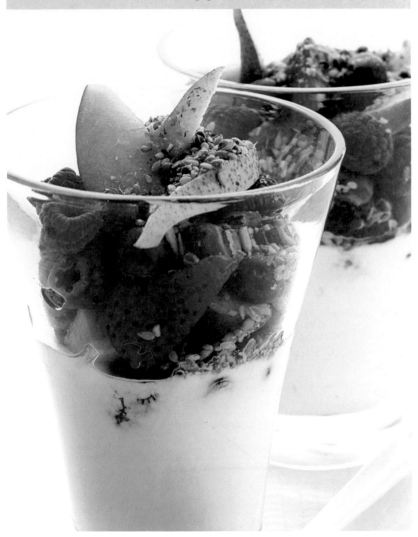

COGNITIVE DECLINE

The prospect of memory loss or a slowing down of mental function in old age is a concern many of us share. Studies show the increase in degenerative brain conditions such as Alzheimer's disease and dementia. While our brains naturally shrink as we age, with Alzheimer's this rate of shrinkage is significantly increased. Yet there is much you can do to reduce your risk of accelerated decline and the sooner you take action the better.

On the list below, tick the symptoms that apply to you on a regular basis:
- ☐ difficulty concentrating
- ☐ finding it harder to do mental arithmetic
- ☐ people pointing out that you repeat yourself
- ☐ finding it harder to remember recent events
- ☐ difficulty remembering people's names
- ☐ feeling mentally tired
- ☐ easily confused by matters you used to take in your stride
- ☐ increasingly losing belongings
- ☐ finding it harder to learn new things

If you ticked three or more symptoms, you may be experiencing memory decline. As well as following the dietary recommendations and supplement suggestions provided here, you may wish to seek additional support from a practitioner who may be able to identify underlying imbalances contributing to your signs and symptoms. By making changes to your diet you may well be able to improve the clarity of your thinking and your alertness.

HEALTHY NEURONS

Your body's ability to maintain cognitive function, a sharpness of mind and a good memory depends significantly on the health of your nerve cells. The efficiency with which messages travel along your nerves and through your brain is, in turn, largely

---

BITE-SIZE SOLUTION

Becoming dehydrated by as little as 1–2% can affect your ability to think clearly and feel refreshed and alert. Aim to drink 1–1½ litres (35–52fl oz/4–6 cups) of water through the day to keep yourself hydrated.

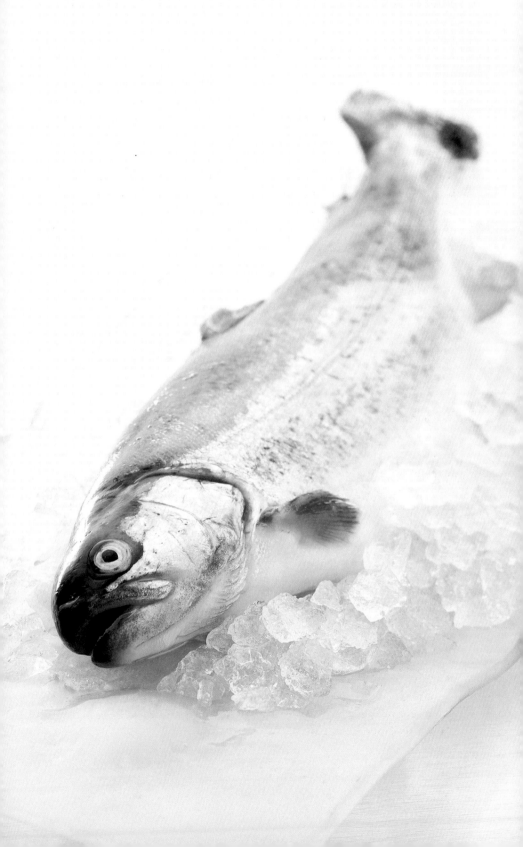

ACTIVE INGREDIENT: CHOLINE

Choline is the raw material for building acetylcholine, a neurotransmitter closely associated with memory function. In Alzheimer's disease there appears to be a reduced ability to convert choline into acetylcholine within the brain.

Choline has also been shown to improve the function of the brain following a stroke. However, like many vital brain chemicals, choline requires efficient methylation to be synthesized from food. Methylation is linked to your homocysteine level: the lower your level, the better you are at methylation and the more able you will be to make phospholipids, such as phosphatidyl choline, and acetylcholine.

So be sure to include plenty of choline in your diet – good sources include organ meats (e.g. liver), fish and eggs. You can also supplement it by taking granules or capsules of lecithin (which contains a phospholipid derived from soya, sunflower or eggs), which are available from health shops. You can sprinkle the granules onto your food or add to juices and smoothies. Take a tablespoon of lecithin granules daily or one 1000mg capsule.

There are other phospholipids that are important for brain function and memory – notably phosphatidyl serine (PS), which is found in fish. Another is DMAE, which acts as a building block for choline and is available as a supplement.

The following recipes contain a source of choline:

BREAKFASTS: Scrambled Eggs on Rye with Leeks and Mushrooms (page 114); Poached Eggs with Asparagus (page 118)

LIGHT MEALS: Chicken Liver and Antipasto Salad (page 131); Beef Fajita with Salsa baked-potato topping (page 124–5)

MAIN MEALS: Frittata (page 142); Fish Soup Provençale (page 138); Herbed Rice Salad with Salmon (page 126)

dictated by the condition of your brain cells, or neurons, and the protective myelin sheath surrounding each of them.

In some conditions involving cognitive decline, damaged proteins build up in neurons and kill them off. However, many other factors influence the health of our neurons. These include: oxidative stress and a lack of antioxidants; reduction in blood supply and oxygen; glycation (damage by excess sugar); damage by toxins; high homocysteine and poor methylation; and a deficiency in the building blocks – omega 3 fats and phospholipid fats – required for cell walls and sheaths.

In addition, levels of certain neurotransmitters are important – in particular our memory neurotransmitter, acetylcholine. Low levels of acetylcholine are associated with Alzheimer's.

HOMOCYSTEINE

High levels of homocysteine (*see also* page 34) have been associated with cognitive decline, memory loss and the risk of developing Alzheimer's, as well as low mood and depression. It appears that high levels lead to a faster rate of destruction of brain cells. You can ask a qualified nutritionist to measure your homocysteine. As we age our levels of homocysteine do rise and we are less able to absorb vitamin B12. Therefore, it is particularly important to check our levels as we age.

Some of us are genetically prone to higher homocysteine levels and consequently need more B vitamins. You can undertake genomic profiles through a qualified nutritionist to determine if you have this genetic predisposition. This will influence the type of supplementation you need and the amount. The easiest way to lower your homocysteine is to take B-vitamin supplements – particularly folic acid, B6 and B12. Ensuring your diet is rich in B vitamins is also crucial as we age. Good sources of B vitamins are whole grains, fish, lentils, most vegetables, wheatgerm and sunflower seeds (*see also* table, page 65).

You can also help optimize your homocysteine levels by making certain changes to your lifestyle. Smoking, drinking coffee and stress can all raise homocysteine, while exercise can naturally improve your level.

The importance of B vitamins in cognitive function is also linked to their role in the production of acetylcholine and phospholipids such as phosphatidyl choline and phosphatidyl serine (*see* box, opposite), which combine with EFAs to make cell membranes. In addition B vitamins such as B12 and folate are essential for oxygen delivery to the brain.

ANTIOXIDANTS

Your brain is rich in fats (*see* page 42), primarily essential fats such as DHA and phospholipids, which are abundant in the protective myelin sheath around each neuron. Essential fats are vulnerable to damage from oxidants, which can arise from many dietary and lifestyle factors including burnt and/or fried foods, processed foods, smoking, trans fats, sugar, environmental pollutants and alcohol. The result is damage to cells, thereby making the body more prone to degeneration, accelerating the ageing process, which includes a decline in nerve health and brain cell function. It is important that you include a high intake of antioxidants to protect the brain from this type of damage. Antioxidants work together to disarm oxidants and the best way to get them is through the food you eat. There is a range of key antioxidants to include daily. These are:

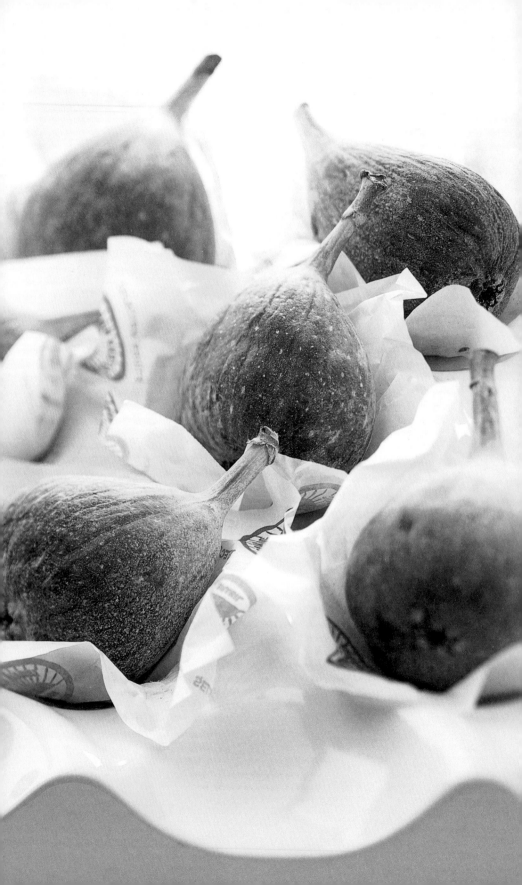

- vitamins A, C and E
- alpha lipoic acid, which protects acetylcholine associated with memory
- glutathione
- N-acetyl cysteine (NAC), which improves methylation and thereby also helps to reduce homocysteine

However, there are many other protective phytonutrients (nutrients present in fruits and vegetables), so include a variety of fresh, organic produce daily. Fruits and vegetables rich in anthocyanidins (e.g. berries and beetroot) appear particularly important. Other foods rich in potent antioxidants include green tea (rich in catechins) and cocoa (a source of epicatechin). See the list of antioxidant-rich foods on page 182 for more details.

AIR SUPPLY

We take on average 26,000 breaths a day. Yet one of the side effects of our sedentary lifestyles and high stress is less effective breathing.

The brain uses up a massive 20% of the oxygen in our body at any given time and any reduction in this can have profound effects on our ability to think clearly and function optimally.

Breathing through the nose and making full use of the diaphragm improves oxygen flow to the body and brain. It also helps to stimulate the vagus nerve to activate the parasympathetic nervous system, which in turn has a calming effect on the body. By learning to breathe correctly we can help ourselves to feel more rejuvenated, refreshed and alert.

RECIPES TO COMBAT AGE-RELATED COGNITIVE DECLINE

BREAKFASTS: Yogurt Fruit Bowl (page 114); Nut and Seed Muesli (page 120); Cinnamon Chia Granola (page 118)

LIGHT MEALS: Mackerel Pâté (page 126); Chicken Liver and Antipasto Salad (page 131)

MAIN MEALS: Prawn and Sea Vegetable Salad with Chilli Lime Dressing (page 131); Grilled Mackerel with Coriander Pesto (page 147); Grilled Rainbow Trout (page 145); Salmon Rolls (page 147); Turmeric and Tamarind Glazed Salmon (page 144)

DESSERTS: Apricot Ice Cream with Pistachios (page 166); Walnut Oat Crumble (page 170)

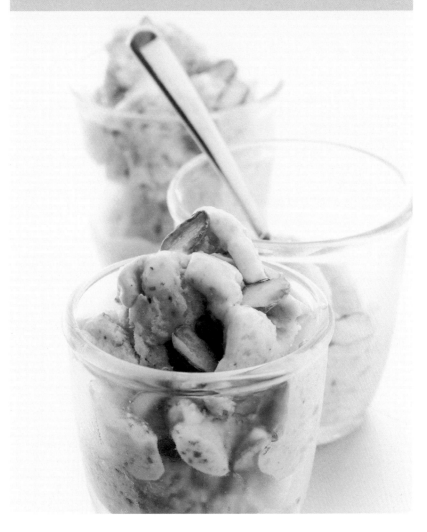

DEPRESSION

**All too often, underlying imbalances in the body that can trigger
or worsen depression are not taken into account when treating
the condition. Here we explore dietary methods that can help you
to overcome depression and take back control of your emotional
well-being.**

Look at the list below and tick any symptoms that sound familiar – answer honestly:

- ☐ feeling depressed or sad
- ☐ feeling low in the mornings
- ☐ you often feel like crying
- ☐ insomnia
- ☐ wanting to be alone or away from contact with others
- ☐ you regularly experience anxiety
- ☐ lack of motivation for and pleasure from activities you usually enjoy
- ☐ poor concentration
- ☐ difficulty making decisions
- ☐ poor appetite or lack of interest in food
- ☐ binge-eating
- ☐ feeling unloved or unwanted
- ☐ tiredness
- ☐ decreased sexual energy (libido)
- ☐ feelings of worthlessness and hopelessness
- ☐ physical symptoms that do not respond to treatment, such as headaches, digestive disorders and chronic pain

If you ticked five or more of the above symptoms you may be suffering from a degree of depression.

Mood disorders are notoriously difficult to categorize and deal with, because they can be triggered by countless different factors. It is clear that the physical and

---

BITE-SIZE SOLUTION

If you are a regular consumer of caffeine, recreational drugs, alcohol or sugar you may benefit from additional tyrosine, which can be rapidly depleted by these stimulants. Good food sources include fish, soya products, poultry, meat, eggs, dairy products, nuts, seeds and oats.

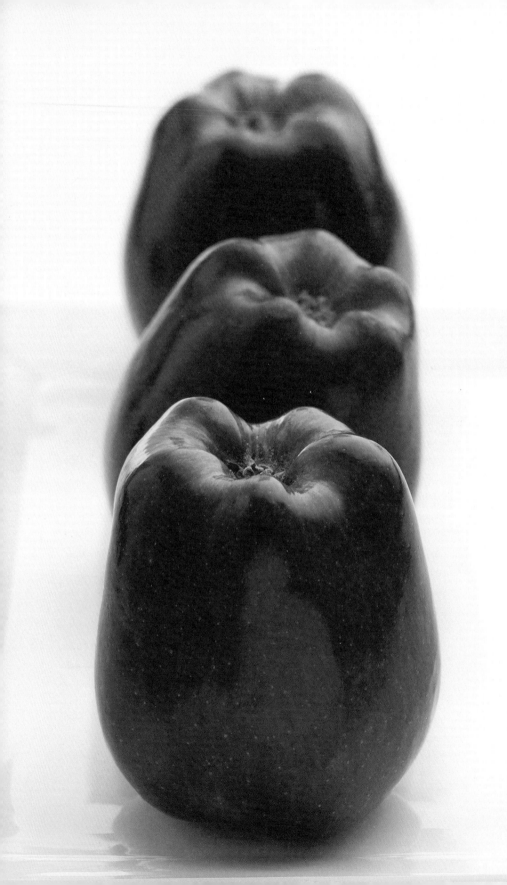

psychological aspects of depression are closely linked. Major life events have an impact on our physical health, which in turn may affect our emotions, particularly in the long term. Therefore, any approach to redressing mood imbalances must take into account both the physical and psychological aspects. Your feelings are not just related to chemistry or the food you have been eating. While the scope of this book is the use of food, lifestyle and dietary changes and supplements to help improve your mood, it is equally important to seek support to help you deal with negative habits, emotions and experiences. If you are suffering from severe depression you should seek specialist help via your doctor.

There are many related factors that can influence your mood which are discussed elsewhere in this book. These include poor sleep (*see* pages 81–5), reduced exposure to daylight (*see* pages 76–80), hormonal imbalances and stress (*see* pages 26–32), and cravings and blood-sugar imbalances (*see* pages 16–25). You may need to read through some of these other sections for further guidance.

NUTRITIONAL DEFICIENCIES

In some cases an imbalance in the brain's chemistry can be related to dietary and nutritional imbalances. Certain nutrients are particularly important in balancing emotions and a reduced level of even one of these may be enough to change your mood for the worse. Key nutrients include amino acids (the building blocks of neurotransmitters), B vitamins, vitamin D, magnesium, zinc and chromium. Ideally, you should consult a qualified nutritionist, who can personalize a dietary programme and supplement plan for you. However, taking a B-vitamin complex formula and a multivitamin and mineral formula to supplement a varied, unprocessed, nutrient-rich diet will be likely to be of benefit.

ESSENTIAL FATS

Numerous studies link depression to low intake of essential fatty acids – particularly omega 3 fats. Increasing your intake of cold-water oily fish may therefore be beneficial. Not only do these provide omega 3 fats but also phospholipids and vitamin D, which are also associated with mood. Eggs are another source of phospholipids and vitamin D. The omega 3 fat EPA appears to be particularly beneficial in combating depression (it can also help relieve aggressive tendencies). Supplementing with at least 1g EPA daily may therefore be beneficial.

See page 182 for a list of foods that are rich sources of essential fats.

ACTIVE INGREDIENT: TRYPTOPHAN

Foods rich in tryptophan, the building block of serotonin, include fish, chicken, turkey, milk, yogurt, cheese, eggs, beans, tofu, bananas, figs, oats, nuts and seeds. By eating these foods with a little carbohydrate, in the form of oats, potato or fresh fruit, you will help the tryptophan to cross the blood–brain barrier and enter the brain. You could also take a 1–3g daily supplement of tryptophan – again, this is best taken with a little fruit juice to aid absorption. As tryptophan can promote sleep, the best time to take it is in the evening. You can also supplement with 5-hydroxytryptophan (5HTP), a precursor to serotonin that increases levels of serotonin in the brain. The recommended dose is around 50–100mg twice a day. Make sure that you also eat plenty of foods rich in vitamin C, B vitamins, magnesium and zinc, as you will need good levels of these nutrients to promote the conversion of tryptophan into serotonin. You may wish to consider taking a supplement with these nutrients included. The following recipes are rich in tryptophan:

BREAKFASTS: Apple Porridge (page 116); Nut and Seed Muesli (page 120); Cinnamon Chia Granola (page 118)

LIGHT MEALS: Chicken Liver and Antipasto Salad (page 131); Root Vegetable Soup (page 136)

MAIN MEALS: Trout with Sunflower Seeds (page 147); Stuffed Vegetables (page 142); Shiitake Chicken (page 153)

DESSERTS: Chocolate Banana Mousse (page 170); Walnut Oat Crumble (page 170)

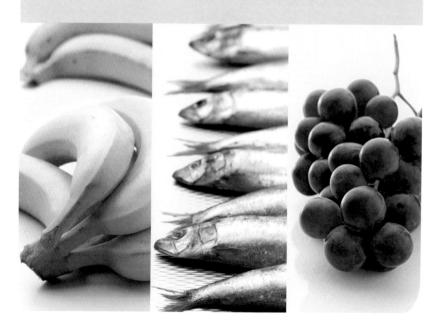

CHROMIUM, MOOD AND BLOOD SUGAR

One of the most crucial factors in balancing out your moods, concentration and energy is maintaining an even blood-sugar level (*see* pages 16–25). The mineral chromium appears to help insulin to function effectively in regulating blood sugar. Chromium may also influence levels of our feel-good neurotransmitter, serotonin. Although chromium is found in foods such as beef, chicken, eggs and fish, you will probably need to take a supplement to obtain an optimal amount. Consider taking 200mcg two or three times a day.

FOOD SENSITIVITIES

Many people find that eliminating certain foods from their diet can have a profoundly positive effect on their mood. See page 57 for a list of foods that most commonly trigger mood changes, along with information on how to identify and eliminate such problem foods from your diet.

HORMONAL BALANCE

A range of hormonal imbalances may be linked to low mood. We have already discussed the action of stress hormones (*see* pages 26–32), as well as the balance of oestrogen and progesterone in women (*see* pages 70–75). However, another hormonal cause of low mood can be an underactive thyroid. The thyroid gland, situated in the base of the throat, produces a hormone called thyroxine, which helps keep the metabolism working at an optimal rate to fuel our body and brain. Low levels of thyroxine can be linked to poor mental function, lethargy, depression and low mood. It can also trigger constipation, skin problems, loss of hair, feeling cold all the time and weight gain. If you are experiencing a number of these symptoms, it may be worth getting your thyroid tested.

However, thyroid function is linked to adrenal health, so a low functioning thyroid gland may be secondary to poor adrenal function. This means you may need to measure both your adrenal and thyroid function. Seek further advice from a nutritionist or healthcare practitioner.

You can support the thyroid gland by boosting your intake of key nutrients such as iodine, selenium, iron, zinc and vitamin A that are required for the conversion of the amino acid tyrosine into thyroxine. See pages 181–3 for a list of the key foods to include in your diet. You may also need to consider eliminating gluten from your diet, because this can trigger autoimmune thyroid conditions.

Some women experience low mood when they are going through the menopause, as a result of falling oestrogen and progesterone levels. Similarly, men with reduced testosterone may suffer a range of symptoms, including loss of libido, erectile dysfunction, poor concentration – and depression. If this profile sounds familiar consider having your hormone levels tested.

TOXIC OVERLOAD

When your body is overloaded – whether that is with too much food, foods that are not nutritious, alcohol, environmental toxins or drugs (prescription or recreational) – you are unlikely to feel well either physically or emotionally. Try following the 7-Day Cleanse programme (*see* pages 52–5) to enhance your body's detoxification processes.

FEEL-GOOD MOOD-BOOSTERS

Many antidepressant drugs act on the brain to prolong the action of feel-good neurotransmitters such as serotonin and noradrenalin in the brain. Yet it is possible to optimize the effect of these neurotransmitters without recourse to medication, purely by introducing changes in your diet and taking the right nutritional supplements.

There are many reasons for low serotonin levels – for example, high cortisol output, low oestrogen and low exposure to daylight. Serotonin is made from the amino acid tryptophan, so by eating foods rich in this nutrient (*see* page 96) you can increase your levels of serotonin.

Noradrenalin is often associated with alertness and motivation. It is derived from the amino acids tyrosine and phenylalanine. Again, as with serotonin, certain vitamins and minerals help convert these amino acids to the neurotransmitters. These include folic acid, vitamin C, magnesium, zinc, iron, copper and manganese. If you feel you are also under a lot of stress, supplementing with tyrosine may be beneficial as adrenalin and noradrenalin are rapidly depleted under long-term stress.

EXERCISE CAN MAKE YOU HAPPY

Studies have shown that regular exercise (30–60 minutes at least three or four times a week) can be as effective as taking antidepressants. Not only does it relieve stress and promote sleep by helping reduce levels of adrenalin and stabilize blood-sugar levels, but if you exercise outdoors you will also expose yourself to sunlight, which can boost levels of vitamin D to the benefit of your mood. However, it is important not to overdo it. Start with a gentle form of exercise that is not too strenuous, such as walking or yoga. For more on the role of exercise in boosting your mood, *see* pages 184–6.

RECIPES FOR LIFTING DEPRESSION

BREAKFASTS: Scrambled Eggs on Rye with Leeks and Mushrooms (page 114); Cinnamon Chia Granola (page 118); Poached Eggs with Asparagus (page 118)

LIGHT MEALS: Baby Spinach, Avocado and Goat's Cheese Salad (page 121); Mackerel Pâté (page 126); Cumin-Spiced Steak with Herb Salsa (page 153); Fish Soup Provençale (page 138); Hot and Sour Soup (page 140)

MAIN MEALS: Scallops with Salsa Verde (page 132); Grilled Rainbow Trout (page 145); Salmon Rolls (page 147); Sesame Stir-Fry (page 149); Mackerel Kedgeree (page 152); Lentils with Spinach (page 154); Spiced Bean Stew (page 157); Grilled Mackerel with Coriander Pesto (page 147); Turmeric and Tamarind Glazed Salmon (page 144)

DESSERTS: Apricot Ice Cream with Pistachios (page 166); Walnut Oat Crumble (page 170); Maca Ice Cream (page 171)

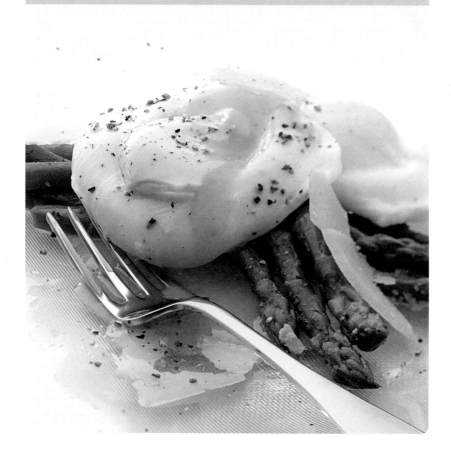

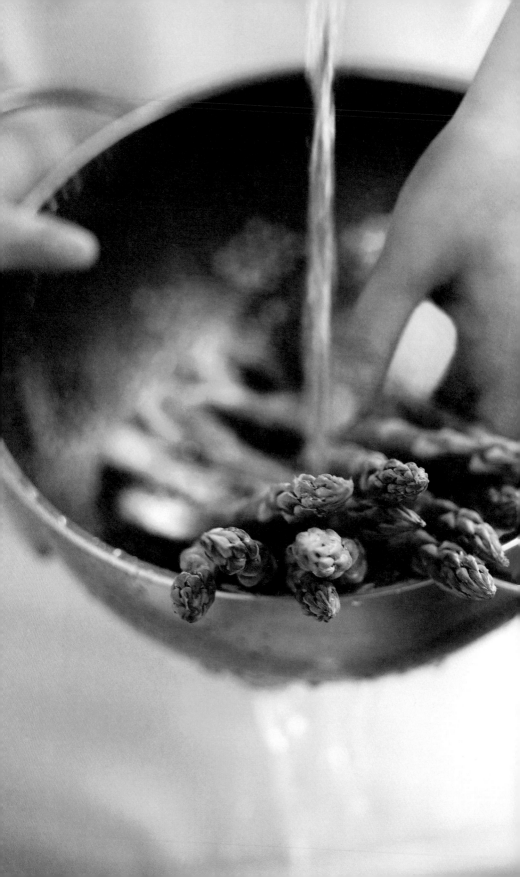

FEEL-GOOD FOOD

You will now be aware of the importance of certain nutrients in helping boost your mood, energy and cognitive function. The dietary recommendations and recipes in this chapter contain these key nutrients as well as avoiding foods that may adversely influence your mood and energy levels. So, by following these recipes you will enrich your diet with unprocessed whole foods, protein, essential fats and low-glycaemic-load carbohydrates to help keep your blood sugar even. You will also take in plenty of B vitamins, antioxidants and minerals to support the production of neurotransmitters in your brain and bolster your energy levels.

However, far from being just essential fuel, food can also be a source of great pleasure and emotional comfort in its own right. The guidelines provided in this chapter give equal emphasis to these valuable aspects of food without losing sight of the impact our dietary choices can have on our health.

FEEL-GOOD DIET

Meals that help maintain good moods, energy levels and general health and well-being are based around a blood-sugar balancing diet rich in nutrients. In this chapter we outline the fundamentals of healthy eating and give a range of recipes that bring these principles together in an appealing and inspiring way.

Dietary strategies aimed at improving your mood – and, at the same time, optimizing all aspects of your physical and mental health – are discussed in detail in the first two chapters of this book. However, we do not always manage to translate these theories into the food on our plates: busy lifestyles, bad dietary habits and the apparent convenience of less healthy foods often take over. Yet by recognizing the powerful impact of eating good food and following some general strategies for boosting your moods and energy levels, it becomes remarkably easy to take the principles outlined in this book with you pretty much anywhere you go.

FEEL-GOOD DIET BASICS

* Start each day with a cup of warm water. You can add lemon juice or fresh ginger (steep the root) if desired. Some people find this helps to stimulate the digestive tract and the bowel.
* Eliminate sugar in all its forms – this includes honey, molasses, agave, high-fructose corn syrup, brown and white sugar, sweeteners.
* Eliminate allergen foods as appropriate, but a trial elimination for one month of gluten and dairy may be particularly beneficial.
* Include slow release, low-glycaemic-load carbohydrates (*see* pages 18–20).
* Include lean protein at each meal and snack – this supplies the amino acids, which are the building blocks of neurotransmitters, and helps stabilize blood-sugar levels. A portion of protein in a meal should measure approximately the size of the palm of your hand.
* Include essential omega 3 fats daily.
* Eat foods high in B vitamins, zinc and magnesium to support methylation.
* Eat fruits and/or vegetables at every meal, making each plate as colourful as possible, so that you are taking in a broad range of beneficial brain-protecting phytonutrients. Some of these should be raw every day – for example, in the form of salads, green juices and smoothies, vegetable crudités and/or marinated vegetables.
* Keep hydrated – drink at least 1.5l (52fl oz/6 cups) filtered water daily.

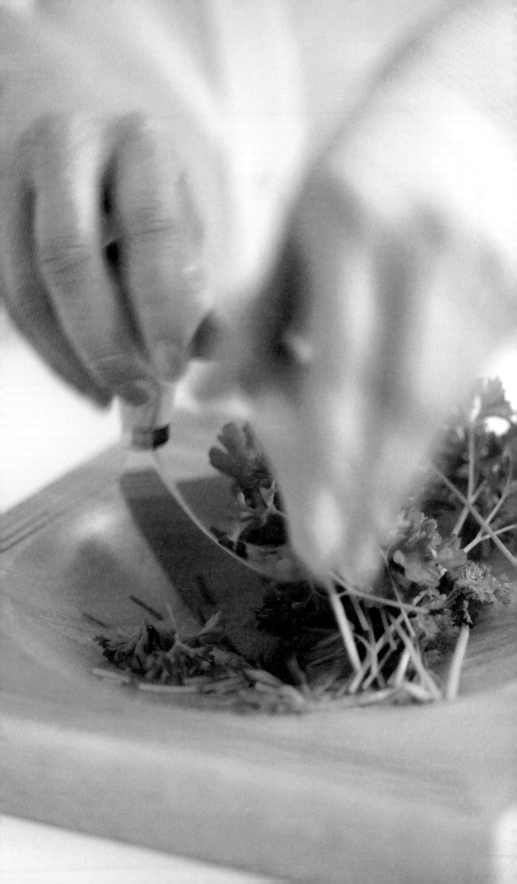

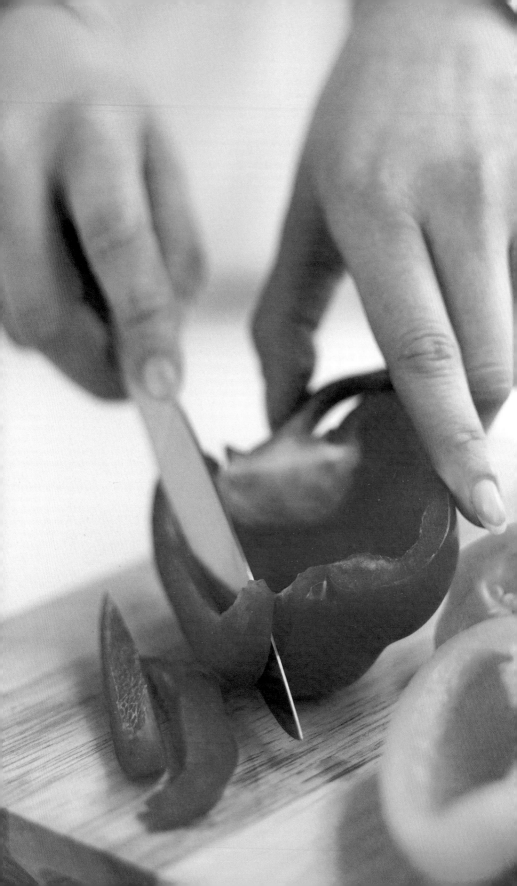

- Avoid stimulants such as caffeine, cigarettes, recreational drugs and alcohol. Switch to decaffeinated options and minimize caffeine to 1–2 cups daily.
- Always eat breakfast and ideally before 10am.
- Snack if you need to keep your blood-sugar levels balanced but do not eat unless you feel hungry.
- Eat organic food wherever possible, to minimize your exposure to antibiotics, pesticides, fertilizers and other chemical residues. Avoid genetically modified foods, as they have not been properly tested and may pose a serious health risk.

PERSONALIZE YOUR PLAN

In addition to the basics listed above, depending on your answers to the questionnaires in the previous chapters you may need to personalize your plan to meet your individual needs:

TO BALANCE YOUR BLOOD SUGAR (SEE PAGES 16–25)

- Consider a blood-sugar support formula that includes chromium, alpha lipoic acid, B vitamins, magnesium and vitamin D3 (*see* page 24).
- Practise mindful eating – slow down and snack regularly.
- Include herbs and plants shown to improve insulin function and/or balance blood-sugar levels such as cinnamon, gymnema, aloe vera, bitter melon, green tea and fenugreek seeds.
- Unless you are trying to gain weight or are doing a lot of exercise, avoid starchy foods like potatoes and grains. Cutting right back on starchy carbs has been found to reduce insulin fluctuations. You will still be taking in enough carbohydrates by eating non-starchy vegetables and fruits.

TO BOOST YOUR LEVELS OF ESSENTIAL FATS (SEE PAGES 38–43)

- Include 1–2 tablespoons ground flaxseed, chia or hemp seed daily – sprinkle over foods or add to smoothies (do not heat).
- Use cold-pressed omega 3 blended oils or flaxseed or hemp oil in salad dressings, drizzled over foods (do not heat).
- Snack on pumpkin, sunflower and sesame seeds or add them to salads.
- Include cold-water oily fish three times a week (e.g. sardines, mackerel, salmon, trout, herring).
- Always use coconut oil for high-temperature cooking and olive oil for lower-temperature cooking.

THE MAKE-UP OF A HEALTHY MEAL

This diagram represents the proportions of fresh vegetables, protein and starch contained in a meal designed to help balance blood-sugar levels. Note that the inclusion of starch in the form of whole grains or starchy vegetables such as potatoes is optional. If you are struggling with blood-sugar levels or trying to lose weight, you should initially cut out all grains and starchy vegetables. Increase your intake of other vegetables and limit fruit to two portions a day.

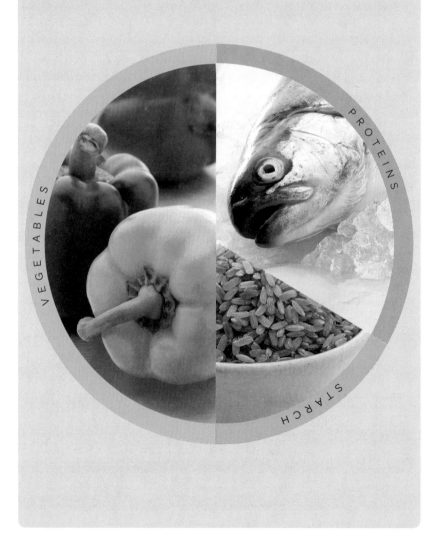

• Consider taking a supplement of 1000mg of EPA/DHA twice a day – look for a blend that also includes omega 6 GLA.

TO OPTIMIZE YOUR DIGESTION AND DETOXIFICATION (SEE PAGES 44–51)
• Consider following the 7-Day Cleanse to support detoxification (*see* pages 52–5).
• Eliminate stimulants such as alcohol, sugar, caffeine and cigarettes completely.
• Take a probiotic – at least 10–20 billion organisms of a broad-spectrum probiotic twice a day.
• Consider including gut-healing support supplements such as L-glutamine, colostrum and vitamin D, as well as digestive enzymes.
• Include more cruciferous vegetables daily (e.g. broccoli, kale, cauliflower, cabbage).
• Include detox foods such as coriander, parsley, dandelion greens, pomegranate and rosemary.
• Take detoxification-supportive supplements such as milk thistle, NAC (N-acetyl cysteine) and vitamin C.
• Combine dietary changes with additional therapies to aid detoxification such as saunas, Epsom salt baths and body brushing (*see* page 53).
• Look for ways to reduce your potential exposure to toxins at home and at work.
• Switch to organic foods where possible.

TO IDENTIFY AND ELIMINATE FOOD SENSITIVITIES (SEE PAGES 56–9)
• Consider taking an IgG food allergy test and, if appropriate, test for coeliac disease.
• Start a food diary to help ascertain likely triggers and your common symptoms. See the full list of common triggers on page 57.
• Eliminate allergens from your diet once you have identified them, choosing suitable alternatives (with the help of a healthcare practitioner) to ensure you are not missing out on important nutrients.
• Take gut-healing supplements before considering a trial reintroduction of any suspect food.

TO TACKLE ONGOING STRESS (SEE PAGES 26–32)
• Seek support from family and friends or look for professional help if necessary.
• Include adaptogenic herbs such as licorice (not with high blood pressure), rhodiola, St John's wort (not with certain medications), maca root, ginseng and cordyceps.
• As stress depletes key nutrients consider including an adrenal supportive formula including magnesium, B vitamins and vitamin C.

- Take gentle exercise daily (*see* pages 184–6) and explore using meditative techniques such as yoga, pilates or prayer.
- Practise mindful eating.
- Find time to relax deeply each day.
- Focus on your breathing.
- Take steps to improve the quality of your sleep (*see* pages 81–5).

EATING OUT

Eating away from home – whether during the working day, business lunches or going out for dinner – is increasingly common. It may seem like hard work to follow the principles of Feel-Good Food when you do not have absolute control over your meals, but it can actually be very easy to do.

For example, breakfast at work or on the run could be a home-made protein bar, a small pot of natural yogurt and a handful of nuts or seeds. A good takeaway lunch might be: salad with plenty of protein (e.g. tuna, chicken, cottage cheese or egg); sushi; bean salad; soup containing protein such as meat or fish (keep your own rice, oat or rye crackers at your desk to have with it); or a bag of raw vegetables with cooked chicken, cottage cheese or hummus.

If you are going out for an occasional meal, you could just enjoy it: choose whatever you fancy from the menu and make the most of a rare treat. However, if you want to follow the recommendations in this book strictly, or you have to eat out regularly, here are some suggestions to bear in mind when selecting your meal:

- Choose a light starter, such as a herb salad or a non-creamy soup.
- Go for a simple main course or ask for it to be cooked plainly – for example, baked chicken without a rich sauce.
- Order plenty of fresh, lightly cooked vegetables or a large salad to go with your main dish; explain that you would like to have more vegetables than potatoes or rice.
- If you order a dessert, share it with someone or just choose a fruit salad.
- Order a peppermint tea instead of coffee – this will not only help your digestion but also refresh your palate.
- Start with a large glass of mineral water, then, if you are drinking wine, alternate a glass of wine with a glass of water, or drink a spritzer (white wine with soda water).

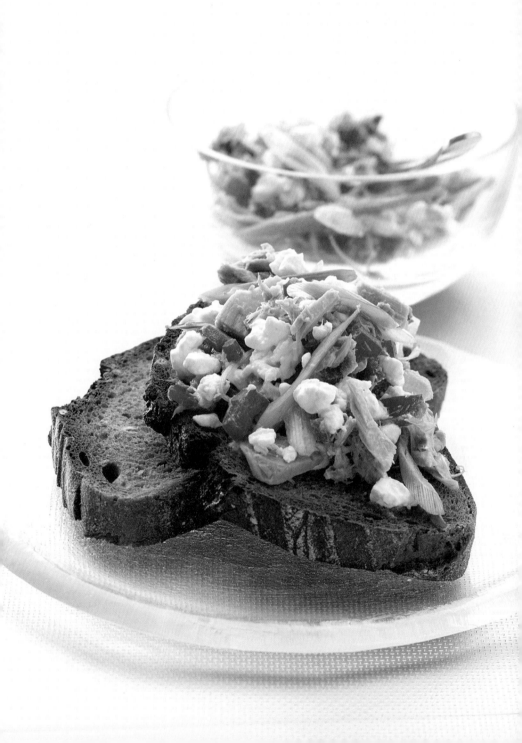

PANTRY

By focusing on the quality of your food rather than on the number of calories or quantity, you will find not only that you will keep those excess pounds at bay but you will significantly improve your mood and energy levels. Therefore, when thinking about foods to stock in your house concentrate on unprocessed, real food. Make fresh vegetables, fruits, whole grains, beans, pulses, nuts and seeds as well as good-quality lean protein central to your diet.

NATURAL SEASONINGS: CONDIMENTS, HERBS AND SPICES

Natural seasonings such as herbs and spices stimulate not only your taste buds but also, in many cases, your body's health systems. Here's what to keep in your kitchen:

Tamari, gluten-free soy sauce (low-sodium brands are also available) – great for flavouring without added fats or sugars.

Seaweed and seaweed flakes – a useful source of iodine for thyroid function and metabolism as well as aiding detoxification.

Chilli pastes and hot pepper sauces – for flavour and stimulating circulation.

Tahini and nut butters – use to enrich sauces and as a spread for crackers.

Sea salt – a useful source of minerals, but use it sparingly.

Fresh ground black pepper – get a grinder and use liberally over foods for flavour.

Spices – keep a range of dried spices to hand: turmeric, cumin, coriander, whole chilli peppers and chilli flakes. Blended spices can liven up meals quickly and cheaply and provide a range of health benefits.

Fresh herbs – use liberally as they have many health-promoting properties and add wonderful flavour to dishes.

Home-made stock – bone broth is a well-known healing food rich in collagen and is also a great base for soups and stews: make your own or use organic fresh stock in pots or low-sodium stock cubes and powders.

Lemon and lime juice and vinegars – use to flavour salads or steamed vegetables; they improve digestion by stimulating stomach acid, as well as helping to lower the glycaemic response of foods they accompany.

OILS

The best oils for cooking are those that remain stable at high temperatures and therefore do not break down into harmful fats. For this reason coconut oil is recommended for cooking in the recipes throughout this book. For lower-temperature cooking, or if you can't get coconut oil, olive oil is a healthy alternative and contains anti-inflammatory and antioxidant phytochemicals. Buy extra virgin oil where possible. Walnut oil is a good option for salad dressings and contains omega 3 fats. Do not cook with cold-pressed seed oils such as flaxseed and hempseed, as they are very sensitive to heat. Instead add them to smoothies, dressings, dips and cold sauces.

NUTS AND SEEDS

Keep a selection of nuts and seeds in your pantry for snacking as well as using in recipes. They are rich in protein, healthy fats and minerals. Buy raw or lightly toasted nuts rather than salted nuts and those fried or roasted in oil. Stick with one or two handfuls for a snack a day. Pumpkin, sunflower, sesame, hemp and flax seeds are all high in fibre, minerals, protein and essential fats. They can be sprinkled over dishes or ground up and added to smoothies.

GO ORGANIC

Where possible choose organic options. Look for animal products that are pasture raised, grass fed and antibiotic and hormone free. Stick to smaller cold-water fish and sustainably farmed fish to reduce mercury load and presence of dioxins. Keeping your diet as clean as possible is crucial for healthy brain function. Sign up to an organic box scheme and try to buy seasonal, local foods where possible.

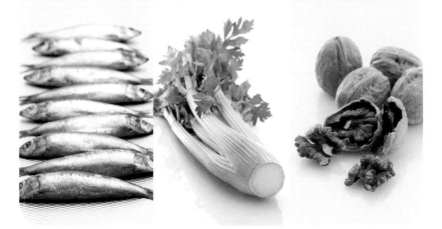

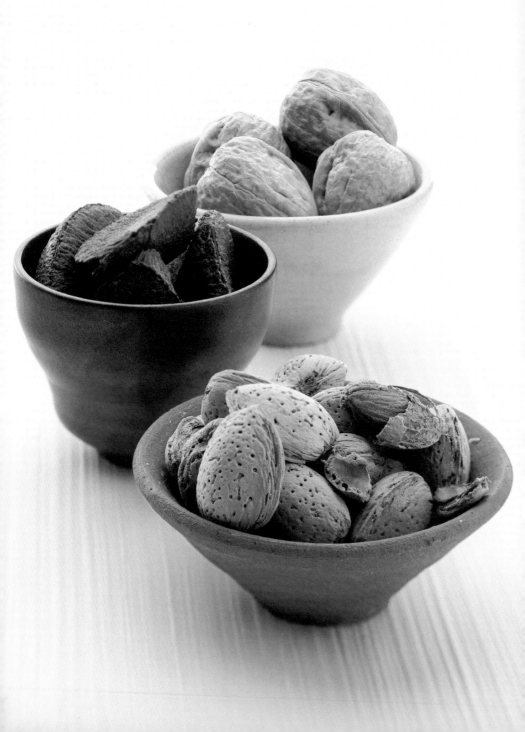

DRINKS

Keeping hydrated through the day is not only great for your brain and energy levels but will stop you snacking constantly too. Always have a glass of water (filtered, if possible) to hand and sip regularly: aim for 1–1.5l (35–52fl oz/4–6 cups) a day. Other healthy drinks include herbal teas, especially peppermint, which may aid concentration, and coconut water, which is rich in hydrating electrolytes. Green tea is another good option. It is rich in antioxidants and an amino acid called theanine, which may aid concentration and focus.

Recent research suggests that coffee may reduce the risk of developing Alzheimer's or dementia. However, too much can upset blood-sugar levels and can make you jittery. Either limit your coffee (and regular tea) intake to 1–2 cups a day, or seek out alternatives such as those made from dandelion root, chicory etc. Watch the labels, though, especially if you are trying to avoid gluten, as many coffee substitutes contain barley and rye.

Avoid fruit juices, squash, soft drinks and soda, even those products labelled sugar free. If you do want to include juices and smoothies, make your own. Focus on vegetable juices rather than fruit juices, and accompany them with a handful of seeds, to avoid upsetting blood-sugar levels. Turmeric is a wonderful anti-inflammatory spice and can be added to smoothies and shakes – simply blend almond or coconut milk with a frozen banana and some vanilla and 1 teaspoon turmeric. Look at our other suggestions for green juices and smoothies in the 7-Day Cleanse section (*see* pages 52–5).

BREAKFASTS

For optimum brain function breakfast is a must. In fact, it really is the most important meal of the day. Glucose is the primary fuel source for the brain, but supply needs to be kept balanced throughout the day. Blood-glucose levels are generally at their lowest after a night of fasting, so eating well in the morning is vital to replenish energy stores.

At breakfast it's important to have some protein, such as meat, fish, yogurt, nuts and seeds or eggs. This makes the meal satisfying and prevents your blood-sugar levels from plummeting soon afterwards (*see* pages 16–25). Breakfast is also the ideal time to sneak in some essential fats, whether it's a portion of oily fish, omega-enriched eggs, or a handful of flaxseed or chia seeds. If you don't feel hungry or are short of time in the morning, you will find many of these recipes are quick and easy to prepare, and can be taken with you to eat on the morning commute or at your desk.

YOGURT FRUIT BOWL *[right]*

Serves 1

Live natural yogurt is packed with healthy bacteria to support digestive health, as well as being a good source of protein to help balance blood-sugar levels. Add some seasonal fruit but opt for low-GL fruit such as berries, apples, plums, peaches, apricots, nectarines and citrus fruits.

250ml (9fl oz/1 cup) natural yogurt
  or soya yogurt
1 serving of chopped fruit, such as
  1 apple or 1 pear, or 80g (2¾oz)
  mixed berries
1 tbsp ground mixed seeds, such as
  sunflower, pumpkin, flaxseed,
  sesame and hemp
½ tsp ground cinnamon

Put the yogurt into a bowl and top with the fruit. Mix the seeds with the cinnamon and sprinkle over the top.

SCRAMBLED EGGS ON RYE WITH LEEKS AND MUSHROOMS

Serves 2

Creamy, soft eggs on rich rye toast with a side serving of leeks and mushrooms makes a satisfying protein-packed breakfast. For additional protein and a source of omega 3 fatty acids, add some chopped smoked salmon to the eggs while cooking.

4 eggs
sea salt and freshly ground black
  pepper
1 tbsp coconut oil

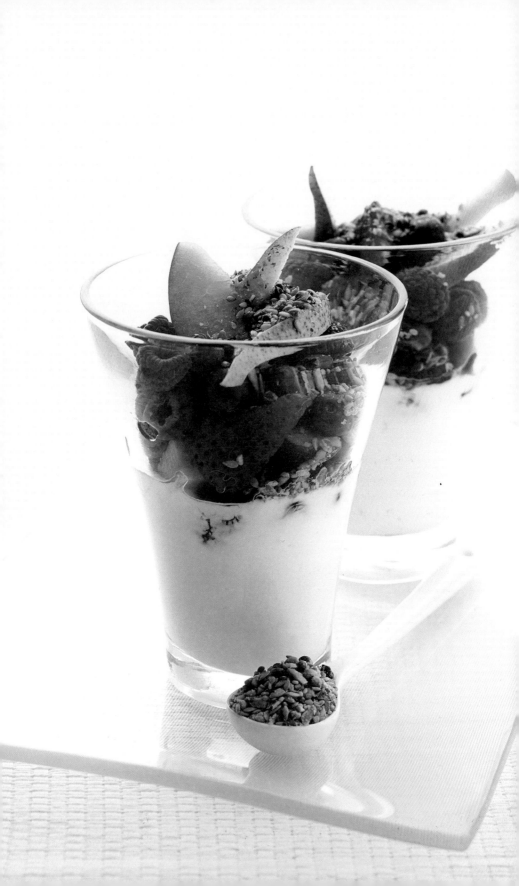

1 large leek, finely sliced

8 chestnut mushrooms, sliced

1 tbsp chopped parsley

2 slices of whole-grain rye bread,
    toasted and lightly buttered

Beat the eggs in a bowl, season to taste
and set aside.

Heat half the oil in a large frying pan,
add the leek and mushrooms and sauté
gently for 5 minutes, or until softened.
Sprinkle over the parsley and divide the
mixture between warmed serving plates.

Heat the remaining oil in the pan over
a very low heat and add the eggs. Stir
constantly until just cooked. Place a slice
of toast on each plate and top with the
scrambled eggs.

APPLE PORRIDGE [below]

Serves 1

A wonderful warming breakfast. Oats
contain plenty of soluble fibre and
slow-releasing carbohydrate to make a
sustaining dish.

50g (1¾oz/½ cup) porridge oats

200ml (7fl oz/scant 1 cup) milk or
    soya milk

1 apple, grated

1 tsp ground cinnamon

2 tsp ground flaxseed

Put the oats into a saucepan with the
milk and 250ml (9fl oz/1 cup) water.
Heat gently for 3–5 minutes, stirring
constantly, until the oats have thickened.

Stir in the apple and cinnamon,
sprinkle over the ground flaxseed and
serve immediately.

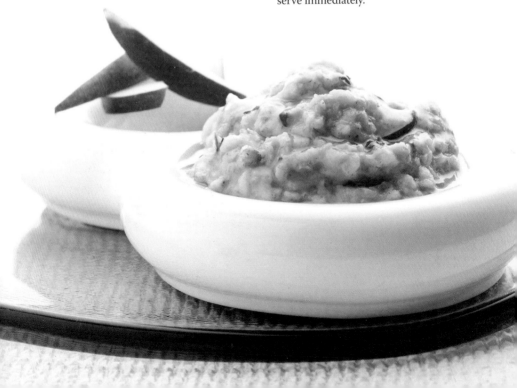

BERRY BRAIN SMOOTHIE

Serves 1

A nutrient-packed smoothie that makes a quick and easy breakfast. Berries are packed with antioxidant phytochemicals that help to protect the brain cells, neurotransmitters and the essential fats in the cell membranes from free-radical attack. Lecithin is an excellent source of phospholipids, which are useful for improving cognitive function.

150g (5½oz) mixed berries, fresh or
    frozen
4 tbsp natural yogurt or soya yogurt
1 scoop vanilla protein powder
1 tsp ground flaxseed
2 tsp omega 3·6·9 oil
2 tsp lecithin granules

Simply place all the ingredients in a blender with 200ml (7fl oz/scant 1 cup) water and blend until smooth. Add a little more water if necessary to reach your preferred drinking consistency.

BUCKWHEAT CRÊPES

Serves 2

Buckwheat is a gluten-free grain rich in tryptophan, the precursor to serotonin, our feel-good neurotransmitter. It also provides plenty of magnesium – an important calming mineral – meaning these crêpes are perfect as an evening snack as well as for breakfast. Serve them with fruit or as a savoury option with cottage cheese, meat or fish.

150ml (5fl oz/scant ⅔ cup) milk or
    soya milk
100g (3½oz/¾ cup) buckwheat flour
a pinch of sea salt
1 egg
coconut oil, for frying

Mix the milk and 150ml (5fl oz/scant ⅔ cup) water together in a jug. Put the flour and salt in a mixing bowl and add the egg. Beat the egg into the flour, adding the milk and water mixture a little at a time to make a batter. Leave for at least 1 hour if possible.

Lightly oil a frying pan and heat it well. Put a tablespoon of batter into the pan and roll it around to the edges. Cook it until the crêpe is golden, then turn over to cook the other side. Repeat with the remaining batter. Serve hot with toppings of your choice.

CINNAMON CHIA GRANOLA

Makes enough for 4 servings

Bake up a batch of this granola and store it in an airtight container for a quick and healthy snack or breakfast. Chia seeds are an excellent source of omega 3 essential fats important for healthy cell membranes and neurotransmitter function.

115g (4oz/heaped 1 cup) porridge
    oats
2 tbsp chia seeds
30g (1oz/¼ cup) shelled hemp seeds
60g (2¼oz/½ cup) sunflower seeds
60g (2¼oz/½ cup) pumpkin seeds
2 tsp ground cinnamon
2 tbsp honey
2 tbsp coconut oil, melted
3 tbsp apple juice

Preheat the oven to 160°C (325°F/gas 2–3). Line a baking tray with non-stick parchment paper.

Combine the oats, seeds and cinnamon in a bowl and stir. In a separate bowl, mix together the honey, oil and apple juice. Stir the honey mixture into the oats and mix thoroughly to coat the dry ingredients.

Spread the mixture onto the baking tray and bake for 45–50 minutes until golden and crisp. Stir occasionally during cooking. Allow to cool completely before serving or storing.

POACHED EGGS WITH ASPARAGUS *[right]*

Serves 2

A delicious quick and easy breakfast. Asparagus is a good source of B vitamins, iron and copper –important cofactors needed for the production of neurotransmitters in the brain.

20 asparagus spears, trimmed
4 eggs
knob of unsalted butter
Parmesan cheese (optional)
freshly ground black pepper

Steam the asparagus spears for 3–4 minutes until tender. Meanwhile, bring a pan of water to the boil, then reduce to a simmer and poach the eggs for 3–4 minutes. Remove the eggs with a slotted spoon and drain on kitchen paper.

Divide the asparagus between plates, dot with butter and lay two poached eggs on top of each asparagus bundle. Scatter over a little Parmesan, if using, and season well with black pepper.

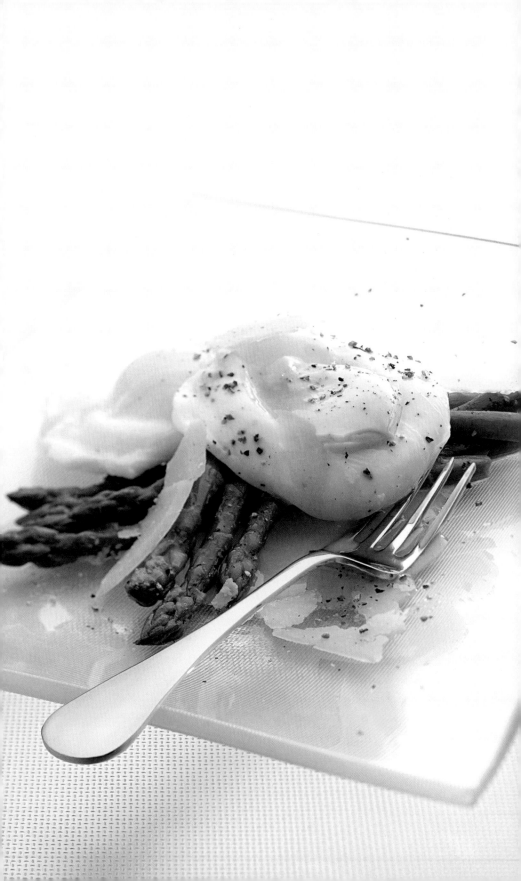

NUT AND SEED MUESLI

Serves 1

This muesli takes seconds to prepare, but you could also make up a large batch for the week and store in an airtight container for ease.

50g (1¾oz/½ cup) porridge oats
½ tbsp oat bran
½ tbsp sunflower seeds
½ tbsp pumpkin seeds
½ tbsp chopped Brazil nuts
½ tbsp chopped almonds
½ tbsp unsweetened coconut flakes
½ tbsp sultanas or raisins (optional)
2 tsp ground flaxseed
milk, soya milk or natural yogurt,
   to serve
1 handful of mixed berries, to serve
   (optional)

Place all the ingredients in a bowl, mix, and store in an airtight container in a cool place. Alternatively, cover an individual serving with water, stir, then place in the fridge overnight. Serve with milk or natural yogurt and some mixed berries, if liked.

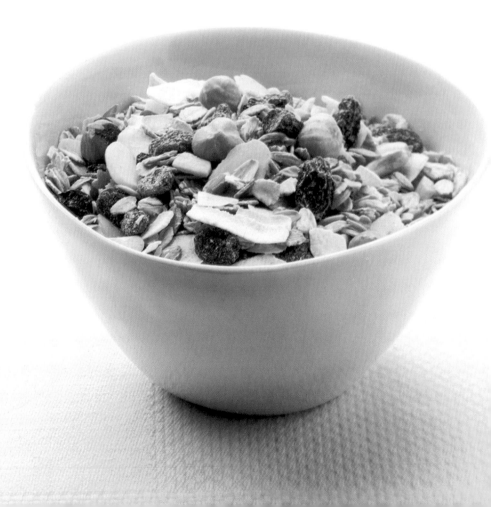

LIGHT MEALS

The following recipes are ideal as a light meal or lunch and are based around energizing proteins, healthy fats and plenty of antioxidant-rich vegetables. Avoid carbohydrate-based meals at lunchtime, as they are more likely to cause fluctuations in blood-sugar levels, resulting in mid-afternoon energy dips that may adversely affect your focus, mood and concentration.

BABY SPINACH, AVOCADO AND GOAT'S CHEESE SALAD

Serves 4

Spinach is a nutrient-packed leafy green providing plenty of B vitamins, magnesium and iron. For a dairy-free option add chunks of cooked tofu or hard-boiled egg. This salad includes plenty of healthy fats from the avocado and walnuts.

**1 ripe avocado, peeled, pitted and
    coarsely diced**
juice of ½ lemon
350g (12oz) baby spinach
200g (7oz) cherry tomatoes, halved
1 small red onion, chopped
150g (5½oz) goat's cheese, crumbled
**115g (4oz/heaped ¾ cup) toasted
    chopped walnuts**
**Creamy Vinaigrette or Sweet and
    Tangy Vinaigrette (*see* page 159)**

Place the avocado in a bowl and drizzle over the lemon juice. Combine the spinach, cherry tomatoes, onion, goat's cheese and toasted walnuts in a bowl. Just before serving add the avocado and pour over the vinaigrette. Mix well and serve immediately.

WARM CHICKEN AND NOODLE SALAD

Serves 2

A delicious gluten-free stir-fry (tamari is a Japanese soy sauce made without wheat). Instead of chicken try using firm tofu or large prawns.

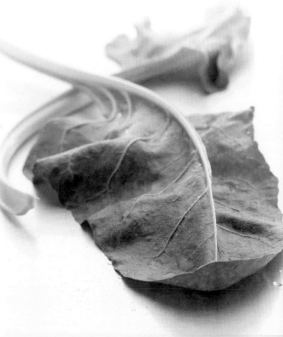

200g (7oz) rice noodles

2 tbsp coconut oil

1 garlic clove, crushed

½ red onion, chopped

4 baby corns, chopped

2 carrots, cut into julienne strips

2 tbsp shredded white cabbage

1 handful of mangetout

250g (9oz) skinless chicken breast,
    cut into strips

1 tbsp sesame oil

2 tbsp tamari soy sauce

2 tbsp mirin

juice of 1 lime

1 handful of coriander, chopped

Cook the noodles according to the
packet instructions. Drain, rinse in cold
water and place in a serving bowl.

Heat half the coconut oil in a wok
or large frying pan and add the garlic
and onion. Sauté for 1 minute. Add the
vegetables and toss until wilted. Add the
mixture to the noodles.

Put the remaining oil in the pan and
stir-fry the chicken in the wok until it
is cooked through. Add the chicken to
the noodles and toss together with the
sesame oil, tamari, mirin, lime juice
and coriander.

MEDITERRANEAN CHICKEN SALAD [right]

Serves 2

Chicken is a good source of protein and
rich in nutrients, including niacin, which
may help reduce the risk of Alzheimer's
disease and age-related cognitive decline
(ARCD). It is also a good source of the
amino acid tryptophan needed to raise
mood-boosting serotonin.

2 large handfuls of baby spinach

1 handful of shredded red cabbage

4 spring onions, finely chopped

8 cherry tomatoes, quartered

2 cold roasted chicken breasts, sliced

For the dressing:

1 tbsp olive oil

1 tbsp flaxseed oil

4 basil leaves, torn or chopped

1 tsp coarse-grain mustard

1 tbsp balsamic vinegar

freshly ground black pepper

Divide the spinach, cabbage, spring
onions and tomatoes between two
serving plates, then arrange slices of
roast chicken on top of the vegetables.

Put the dressing ingredients in a jar
and shake well. Pour the dressing over
the chicken and serve.

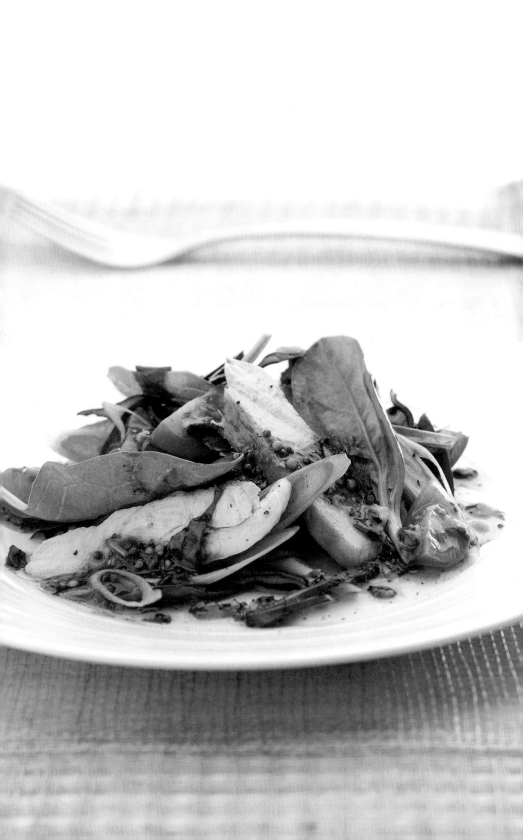

BAKED-POTATO TOPPINGS

Each topping serves 2

A small baked potato makes a quick light meal but make sure you combine it with plenty of protein to keep energy levels high and blood-sugar levels balanced. For a more nutritious option try baking sweet potatoes, which are particularly rich in antioxidants, especially beta-carotene, useful for protecting the brain cells against free radical damage. To cook the baked potatoes, heat the oven to 180°C (350°F/ gas 4), wash and prick the potatoes and put them in the oven on a baking tray for about an hour, depending on the size of the potato. Check whether they are cooked through and soft by pricking them with a skewer. Add a topping of your choice and accompany with a nutrient-dense green salad.

HUMMUS, AVOCADO AND ALFALFA TOPPING *[below]*

4 tbsp ready-made hummus
½ ripe avocado, peeled and pitted
2 handfuls of alfalfa sprouts

Mash the hummus with the avocado and top with alfalfa sprouts.

MUSTARD CHICKEN TOPPING

2 cooked chicken breasts, diced
2 tbsp natural yogurt
1 tsp coarse-grain mustard
freshly ground black pepper
sprouted rocket and/or cress shoots

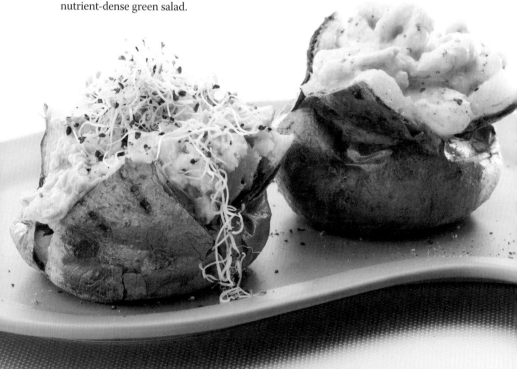

Mix together the chicken, natural yogurt and mustard and season well with black pepper. Top with the rocket and/or cress shoots, which are available at most supermarkets.

BEEF FAJITA WITH SALSA

juice of 1 lime
1 tbsp olive oil
1 garlic clove, crushed
½ tsp ground cumin
½ tsp fajita seasoning
freshly ground black pepper
250g (9oz) beef steak
2 tbsp ready-made salsa

Mix together the lime juice, oil, garlic, cumin, fajita seasoning and season well with black pepper. Pour the mixture over the beef, cover, and marinate for at least 30 minutes.

Heat a frying pan over a high heat and cook the steak for 3–4 minutes on each side. Rest the meat for 10 minutes then slice thinly. Top the potato with the beef and add the salsa.

SPICY PRAWN TOPPING

[below, left]
150g (5½oz) small cooked peeled prawns
1 tbsp natural yogurt
2 tsp low-sugar tomato ketchup
dash of Tabasco sauce
squeeze of lemon juice

Mix together the prawns, yogurt, ketchup and Tabasco sauce. Add a squeeze of lemon juice and stir well.

SMOOTH SALMON TOPPING

1 x 200-g (7-oz) tin pink salmon in spring water, drained
1 tbsp cottage cheese
1 spring onion, finely sliced
1 tbsp chopped parsley
squeeze of lemon juice
freshly ground black pepper

With a fork, mash the salmon with the cottage cheese in a bowl. Add the other ingredients, then season with black pepper and mix well.

MACKEREL PÂTÉ

Serves 2

Simple and quick to prepare, this protein-packed pâté is a great source of omega 3 fats. Use as a topping for oat cakes or rice cakes or as part of a light meal accompanied by a salad. This will keep in the fridge for up to 3–4 days.

115g (4oz) smoked mackerel fillet, broken up into pieces
2 spring onions, chopped
110g (3¾oz) low-fat cream cheese or quark
1 tbsp lemon juice
1 tbsp chopped parsley
1 tbsp chopped dill

Place all the ingredients in a food processor and process until smooth. Chill until needed.

HERBED RICE SALAD WITH SALMON *[below]*

Serves 2–3

Brown rice is a low-GL grain rich in minerals including manganese and selenium – two key nutrients required for antioxidant protection. Tinned salmon is a healthier option than tuna as the canning process removes most of the omega 3 fatty acids in the tuna, and being a larger oily fish it is generally higher in mercury and chemical pollutants. For more of a Mediterranean flavour add some sundried tomatoes and marinated artichokes.

200g (7oz/1 cup) brown rice
3 eggs
3 tomatoes, deseeded and chopped
1 green pepper, chopped

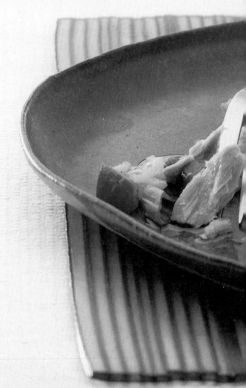

4 spring onions, finely chopped

12 olives, halved

2 tbsp chopped mint

2 tbsp chopped parsley

2 tbsp chopped coriander

1 x 200-g (7-oz) tin salmon or tuna
   in spring water, drained

For the dressing:

2 tbsp capers, chopped

2 tsp Dijon mustard

2 tbsp red wine vinegar

1 tbsp lemon juice

3 tbsp flaxseed oil or omega 3·6·9 oil

sea salt and freshly ground black
   pepper

Cook the rice according to the packet instructions and set aside to cool. Cook the eggs until they are hard boiled and leave to cool.

Put the rice in a large bowl and mix in the vegetables, olives and herbs. Shell the eggs and cut into quarters.

Flake the salmon and add to the rice salad with the eggs. Whisk together the capers, mustard, vinegar, lemon juice and oil and season. Pour the dressing over the salad and toss lightly to serve.

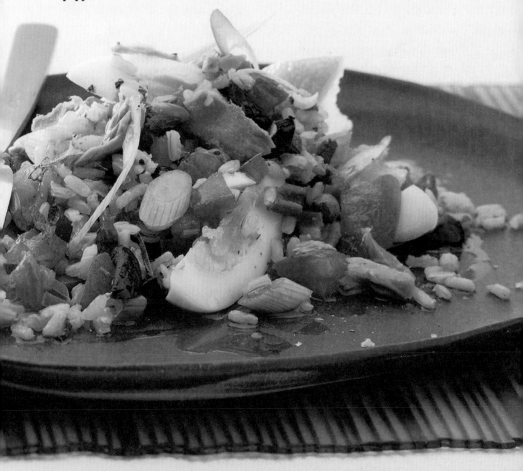

CHICKEN AND MUSHROOM PÂTÉ

Serves 2, or 4 as a starter

This is good for serving as a starter at a dinner party. It also makes a simple, satisfying lunch. Eat with rye or rice crackers as a starter or with a large salad as a meal in itself. You can vary the herbs to suit your taste.

1 cooked chicken breast, shredded
4 medium-sized chestnut mushrooms, roughly chopped
2 spring onions, roughly chopped
50g (1¾oz) cottage cheese
2 tbsp olive oil
1 tsp chopped tarragon, plus sprigs for garnishing (optional)
1 tsp chopped parsley, plus sprigs for garnishing (optional)
sea salt and freshly ground black pepper

Put all the ingredients in a blender, season, and blend until smooth. Alternatively, for a rougher pâté, simply chop the chicken, mushrooms and onion very finely and mix with all the ingredients in a bowl. Put the pâté in the fridge to chill.

If the pâté is for a dinner party, you can serve it in four individual ramekin dishes. Garnish with sprigs of tarragon or parsley, if using, just before serving.

SHREDDED CHICKEN LETTUCE WRAPS WITH WALNUT OIL VINAIGRETTE

Serves 2

A light, low-carb dish using lettuce leaves instead of bread to enclose the filling. Walnut oil is a good source of omega 3 essential fats and provides a wonderful nutty flavour to the dressing.

For the dressing:
2 tbsp sherry vinegar
3 tbsp walnut oil
1 tbsp olive oil
a pinch of sugar
½ tsp Dijon mustard

1 tbsp coconut oil
115g (4oz) mixed mushrooms, sliced
1 garlic clove, crushed
2 roasted chicken breasts, shredded
60g (2¼oz/½ cup) walnut pieces, toasted
6–8 cos lettuce leaves

Whisk together the ingredients for the dressing and set aside.

Heat the oil in a frying pan and sauté the mushrooms and garlic for 3–4 minutes until browned, taking care not to burn the garlic. Place in a bowl with the chicken and walnuts, add the dressing and mix gently. Spoon the chicken mixture into the lettuce leaves and serve immediately.

RED CABBAGE AND FETA SALAD [below]

Serves 2

The sharp taste of red cabbage goes beautifully with the rich feta cheese and sweet apple. Adding the seeds provides additional protein and healthy fats.

½ large red cabbage, finely shredded
150g (5½oz) feta cheese, crumbled
1 apple, diced
2 tbsp shelled hemp seeds
2 tbsp sunflower seeds
4 tbsp Sweet and Tangy Vinaigrette
   (*see* page 159)

Mix together the cabbage, cheese and apple. Sprinkle over the seeds and toss well in the vinaigrette.

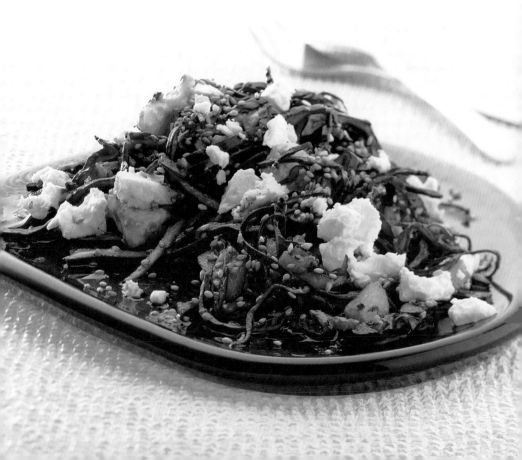

MIXED BEAN AND GOAT'S CHEESE SALAD WITH LEMON OIL DRESSING

Serves 2

This is quick and easy to assemble and ideal as a portable packed lunch. Take the dressing in a separate container and dress just before serving.

For the dressing:
juice of 1 lemon
3 tbsp olive oil
2 tbsp flaxseed oil
1 tbsp honey

1 x 420-g (15-oz) tin mixed beans, drained
1 celery heart, thinly sliced
½ red onion, finely chopped
1 large handful of chopped parsley
1 large handful of chopped mint
1 large tomato, roughly chopped
1 red chilli, deseeded and finely chopped
150g (5½oz) green beans, trimmed and blanched
115g (4oz) goat's cheese, crumbled

Whisk together the ingredients for the dressing and set aside. Mix together all the remaining ingredients in a bowl. Pour over the dressing and toss lightly just before serving.

SPINACH DAHL

Serves 2

Lentils are a good source of protein and soluble fibre, making them useful for stabilizing blood-sugar levels and providing slow-release energy. Add plenty of turmeric to this dish as this potent anti-inflammatory spice has been shown to protect against neurodegenerative diseases such as Alzheimer's. Accompany with steamed greens or a mixed salad.

100g (3½oz/heaped ⅓ cup) red lentils
450ml (16fl oz/scant 2 cups) vegetable stock
1 small onion, grated or very finely chopped
2 garlic cloves, crushed
2 tomatoes, chopped
1 tsp turmeric
1 tsp garam masala
1 red chilli, finely chopped
2 handfuls of young leaf spinach

Put all the ingredients except the spinach in a pan. Bring to a boil, then turn the heat down and simmer for about 20 minutes until the lentils are soft. Stir in the spinach and cook for a minute until wilted.

PRAWN AND SEA VEGETABLE SALAD WITH CHILLI LIME DRESSING

Serves 2

Sea vegetables are rich in many minerals and antioxidants, as well as polysaccharides, which have anti-inflammatory properties. Prawns are a useful source of protein needed for the production of neurotransmitters for healthy brain function.

30g (1oz) mixed sea vegetables, soaked in water for 10 minutes, then drained
2 large handfuls of watercress
1 carrot, cut into julienne strips
1 red pepper, thinly sliced
4 spring onions, thinly sliced
½ cucumber, deseeded and cut into julienne strips
250g (9oz) large cooked prawns

For the dressing:
juice of 2 limes
1 tsp sugar
1 garlic clove, crushed
1 tbsp coriander leaves, chopped
1 tbsp fish sauce

Place all the vegetables in a bowl and toss in the prawns. Whisk together the ingredients for the dressing and drizzle over the salad to serve.

CHICKEN LIVER AND ANTIPASTO SALAD

Serves 2

Liver is a good source of choline, the precursor for our memory neurotransmitter acetylcholine. A lack of choline intake has been linked to memory loss. Try to use organic chicken livers for this dish.

2 large handfuls of bitter salad leaves (such as rocket, watercress or endive)
Creamy Vinaigrette (*see* page 159)
4 marinated chargrilled artichoke hearts, quartered
1 handful of black olives, halved
1 roasted red pepper, sliced
1 tbsp coconut oil
sea salt and freshly ground black pepper
200g (7oz) organic chicken livers, sliced

Put the salad leaves in a bowl and toss with some of the vinaigrette. Divide between plates and top with the artichokes, olives and red pepper.

Heat the oil in a frying pan over a medium heat. Season the livers and sauté for about 2 minutes until they are firm but not hard. Place on top of the salads and drizzle with a little more dressing to serve.

TERIYAKI VENISON SALAD

Serves 2

Like other game meats venison is rich in the amino acids phenylalanine and tyrosine, the precursors required to boost dopamine levels. Dopamine is a neurotransmitter associated with alertness, focus and concentration. Instead of venison you could use beef or lamb fillet.

2 tbsp tamari soy sauce
1 tbsp rice wine
1 tbsp honey
2 garlic cloves, crushed
250g (9oz) venison fillet
1 tbsp freshly ground black pepper
large bag mixed salad greens
100g (3½oz) sugar snap peas

Mix together the tamari, rice wine, honey and garlic. Pour over the venison, cover, and leave to marinate in the fridge for at least 1 hour, or overnight.

Preheat the oven to 200°C (400°F/ gas 6). Remove the venison from the marinade, reserving the marinade. Season the venison with black pepper and sear in a hot frying pan on both sides. Place in the oven for 15 minutes, or until cooked to your liking. Rest for 5 minutes before slicing.

Pour the marinade into a small pan and bring to the boil, then turn down the heat and simmer for about 5 minutes, or until you have a thick, syrupy glaze.

Arrange the salad greens and sugar snap peas on a platter and top with the venison. Drizzle over the marinade.

SCALLOPS WITH SALSA VERDE

Serves 2

Scallops are a great source of protein and they also contain omega 3 essential fats and B vitamins important for brain health. This is a quick and light dish full of Mediterranean flavours. Accompany with a mixed salad.

1 tbsp olive oil
6 scallops, shelled
sea salt and freshly ground black pepper
1 tbsp lemon juice

For the Salsa Verde:
1 handful of parsley
1 handful of basil leaves
1 handful of mint leaves
2 garlic cloves, crushed
2 anchovies
1 tbsp capers
2 tbsp red wine vinegar
1 tsp Dijon mustard
150ml (5fl oz/scant ⅔ cup) olive oil

Drizzle the oil over the scallops and season well.

For the Salsa Verde, put the herbs, garlic, anchovies, capers, red wine vinegar and mustard in a food processor and process until chunky. Slowly add the oil to create a thick dressing.

Heat a frying pan and sear the scallops for 1 minute on each side. Drizzle over the lemon juice and serve immediately with the Salsa Verde on the side.

PUY LENTIL SALAD [below]

Serves 2

Puy lentils are high in fibre and provide plenty of slow-release energy to help satisfy the appetite and avoid mid-afternoon energy slumps. This delicious salad is dressed with a walnut and balsamic vinaigrette to provide plenty of health-promoting omega 3 fats.

250g (9oz/1¼ cups) puy lentils
3 tomatoes, chopped
3 spring onions, finely sliced
6 basil leaves, torn

For the dressing:
3 tbsp balsamic vinegar
½ tsp Dijon mustard
2 tbsp walnut oil
2 tbsp olive oil
sea salt and freshly ground black
    pepper

Place the lentils in a large pan, cover with cold water and bring to the boil. Turn the heat down, cover with a lid and simmer for 15–20 minutes, or until al dente. Drain the lentils and place in a bowl. Add the tomatoes, spring onions and basil leaves.

Whisk together the ingredients for the dressing, pour over the lentil salad and toss lightly to coat.

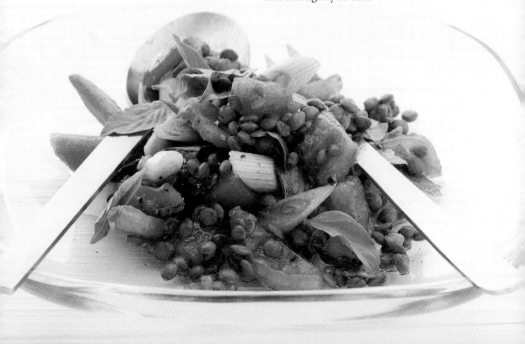

SOUPS

Soups are incredibly nourishing and an ideal way to cram in plenty of nutrient-rich vegetables. Make up a large batch and freeze in portions to make a speedy light meal when time is short. For an energizing lunch accompany soup with some additional protein such as slices of cooked fish, chicken or eggs.

FREEZING

Once cool, all these soups can be frozen in freezable containers for 2–3 months.

CARROT SOUP [right]

Serves 3–4

A hearty, thick soup rich in vitamin C and beta-carotene. These antioxidants are important to help protect the brain cells, neurotransmitters and the essential fats in the cell membranes from free radical attack.

1 onion, chopped
1 garlic clove, chopped
1 tsp olive oil
500g (1lb 2oz) carrots, chopped
2 celery sticks, chopped
½ tsp whole-grain mustard
½ tsp onion powder
½ tsp sea salt
dash of Tabasco
sprigs of fresh thyme
1.25cm (½in) piece of root ginger, peeled and grated
1l (35fl oz/4 cups) chicken or vegetable stock
natural yogurt or soya yogurt
freshly ground black pepper

In a large pan, soften the onion and garlic in the oil for a couple of minutes. Add the carrots, celery, mustard, onion powder, salt, Tabasco, thyme, ginger and stock. Bring to the boil, then turn the heat down, cover with a lid and simmer for 30 minutes. Purée the soup with a hand-held blender or pour into a food processor and blend until smooth. Swirl 1 teaspoon of natural yogurt in each bowl. Season with black pepper and serve.

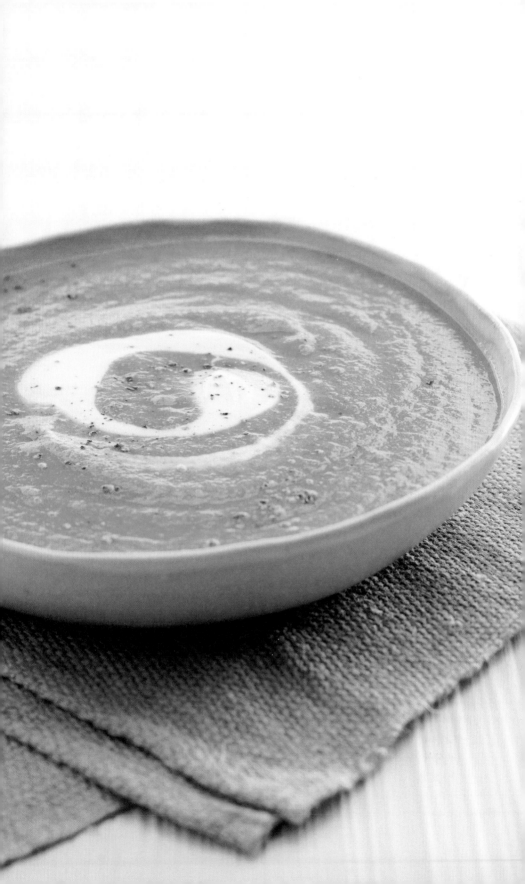

ROOT VEGETABLE SOUP

Serves 4

A wonderful earthy soup making the most of seasonal root vegetables. Adding a can of beans provides additional protein. Vary the vegetables according to season.

250g (9oz) baby carrots, halved lengthways

1 parsnip, cut into small chunks

½ swede, cut into small chunks

1 red onion, cut into wedges

olive oil, for roasting

a pinch of dried chilli flakes

2 tsp ground cumin

sea salt and freshly ground black pepper

1l (35fl oz/4 cups) chicken or vegetable stock

5–6 kale leaves, tough ends trimmed

1 x 400-g (14-oz) tin cannellini beans (optional)

1 small bunch of coriander, chopped

Preheat the oven to 190°C (375°F/gas 5). Arrange all the vegetables except the kale in a large roasting tin. Drizzle over some oil and sprinkle over the chilli flakes and cumin, then season. Toss well and roast for 30 minutes.

Put the stock in a large saucepan and bring to the boil. Add the roasted vegetables, kale and beans, if using, and cook for 5 minutes. Stir in the coriander and serve.

THAI-STYLE NOODLE SOUP *[right]*

Serves 4

This makes a perfect meal in a bowl. If you're having this for lunch include plenty of protein, such as prawns, tofu or cooked chicken, to keep energy levels high throughout the afternoon. Ginger and garlic are wonderful stimulatory spices – great for improving circulation and reducing inflammation.

150g (5½oz) vermicelli rice noodles

1 tbsp coconut oil

2 tsp Thai green curry paste

1 lemongrass stalk, trimmed and finely chopped

2 garlic cloves, finely chopped

2.5cm (1in) piece of root ginger, peeled and finely sliced

250g (9oz) large raw peeled prawns, cooked chicken or cooked tofu

8 baby corns, sliced

8 spring onions, sliced

2 carrots, sliced

12 mangetout, sliced in half lengthways

1 x 400-ml (14fl-oz/1½-cups) tin coconut milk

3–4 kaffir lime leaves

1 handful of coriander, chopped

Cook the rice noodles according to the packet instructions, rinse well with cold water and divide between four large warmed bowls.

Heat the oil in a large frying pan or wok and stir in the curry paste, lemongrass, garlic and ginger. Add 1 tablespoon water.

Toss in the prawns and stir for a few minutes until cooked through. Remove from the pan with a slotted spoon and lay them on the noodles.

Add the vegetables to the pan, stirring them in the spices for a couple of minutes. Pour in the coconut milk and add the kaffir lime leaves. Fill the coconut milk tin with cold water and add to the pan (repeat if you like a slightly thinner soup).

Bring to the boil, then turn the heat down and leave to simmer for 10 minutes, or until the vegetables are cooked. At the last minute, stir in half the coriander.

Ladle the soup evenly over the noodles and prawns and garnish with the remaining coriander.

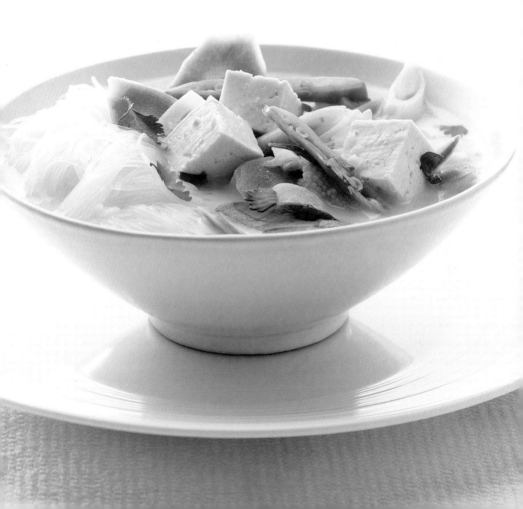

LEEK AND POTATO SOUP

Serves 3–4

Leeks, like garlic and onions, contain many beneficial compounds including flavonoids and sulphur-containing nutrients. They are also a good source of folate, important for lowering homocysteine.

½ onion, chopped
1 garlic clove, crushed
1 tsp olive oil
3 leeks, sliced
1 large potato, chopped
600ml (21fl oz/scant 2½ cups)
   vegetable stock
1 bouquet garni
2 tsp tamari soy sauce
sea salt and freshly ground black
   pepper
natural yogurt or soya yogurt,
   to serve

In a large pan, soften the onion and garlic in the oil for a couple of minutes, then add the leeks, potato and 3 tablespoons of the stock and stir.

Pour in the rest of the stock, add the bouquet garni and season well with the tamari and black pepper. Cover with a lid and leave the soup to simmer for 20–25 minutes until the potato is soft. Pour into a blender and process until smooth. Season to taste and serve swirled with a teaspoon of natural yogurt in each bowl.

FISH SOUP PROVENÇALE

Serves 4

A flavoursome tomato broth forms the basis of this summery, chunky soup. It contains an array of seafood rich in protein and healthy omega 3 fats. Try to use sustainable fish where possible.

2 tbsp coconut oil
2 garlic cloves, crushed
1 fennel bulb, cored and chopped
a pinch of dried chilli flakes (optional)
½ tsp smoked paprika
1 x 400-g (14-oz) tin plum tomatoes
400ml (14fl oz/1½ cups) fish or
   chicken stock
200g (7oz) skinless, boneless firm
   white fish, cut into chunks
200g (7oz) skinless, boneless salmon,
   cut into chunks
100g (3½oz) cooked mussels
100g (3½oz) cooked and peeled
   prawns
1 bunch of flat-leaf parsley, chopped

Heat the oil in a large pan. Add the garlic and fennel cook for 5 minutes until softened. Add the chilli flakes and paprika, then tip in the tomatoes and stock and bubble for 15–20 minutes until thickened slightly. Turn the heat down to a simmer, add the fish and cook for about 5 minutes until it is completely cooked through.

Add the mussels and prawns and heat through. Sprinkle with parsley to serve.

WARMING LAMB SOUP
Serves 4

Rather than using lamb fillet you could add cooked roast lamb with the beans at the end of cooking. Use quality, fresh stock or make your own. Lamb is a rich source of protein, B vitamins and minerals, including iron, zinc and calcium, important for a healthy brain.

1 tbsp coconut oil
sea salt and freshly ground black
    pepper
200g (7oz) lamb neck fillet, trimmed
    and cut into small pieces
1 large onion, chopped
2 garlic cloves, chopped
2 celery sticks, sliced
2 carrots, sliced
2 tsp Worcestershire sauce
1l (35fl oz/4 cups) lamb or chicken
    stock
3–4 thyme sprigs
1 x 400-g (14-oz) tin cannellini beans

Heat the oil in a large saucepan. Season the lamb, then fry for a few minutes until all the pieces are browned. Add the onion and garlic and fry gently for 1 minute. Add the celery and carrots and cook for a further 2 minutes, then add the Worcestershire sauce, stock and thyme. Cover with a lid and simmer for 20 minutes.

Add the beans and heat through. Depending on how you like your soup, you can serve this as it is or purée some or all of it with a hand-held blender or in a food processor.

BEAN AND COURGETTE SOUP WITH PESTO
Serves 3–4

This is a variation on a pistou soup popular in France. Adding beans increases the protein content of the soup to help stabilize blood-sugar levels and keep you feeling alert.

1 onion, sliced
1 tbsp coconut oil
250g (9oz) green runner beans, sliced
2 x 420-g (15-oz) tins haricot beans
2 large courgettes, sliced
1l (35fl oz/4 cups) vegetable stock

For the Pesto:
3 garlic cloves
1 handful of basil leaves, plus extra to
    garnish
3 tomatoes, peeled and chopped
1 tbsp freshly grated Parmesan cheese,
    plus extra to serve
sea salt and freshly ground black
    pepper
1–2 tbsp olive oil

In a large pan, soften the onion in the coconut oil. Add the runner and haricot beans and courgettes and stir for a few minutes. Add the stock and simmer for about 20 minutes, or until the vegetables are cooked.

While the soup is cooking, make the Pesto. Put the garlic, basil leaves, tomatoes and Parmesan in a blender and season with a pinch of salt and freshly ground black pepper. Blend while slowly adding enough olive oil to make a pesto sauce. Check the soup – if it gets too thick, add a little more water.

Just before serving, pour the pesto sauce into the soup and stir well. Serve each bowl of soup topped with some freshly grated Parmesan and a basil leaf.

HOT AND SOUR SOUP

[right]

Serves 4

This is an authentic and deliciously nourishing clear Thai broth with seafood and plenty of flavour. Instead of prawns you could add fish, chicken or tofu. Ideally use home-made fish stock, prepared by boiling fish bones with lemongrass, chilli, kaffir lime leaves and galangal, but if you don't have the time you can buy fresh fish or chicken stock.

1.5l (52fl oz/6 cups) fish or chicken
    stock
2 small red chillies
1 lemongrass stalk, trimmed and
    sliced
2.5cm (1in) piece of root ginger, peeled
    and grated
3 dried kaffir lime leaves
3 slices dried galangal (optional)
2 tsp brown sugar
4 spring onions, sliced
500g (1lb 2oz) large raw peeled prawns
1 tbsp fish sauce
1 tbsp tamari soy sauce
1 tbsp fresh lime juice
sea salt and freshly ground black
    pepper
115g (4oz) enoki mushrooms
1 handful of coriander leaves, chopped

Place the stock in a large pan and bring to the boil. Add the chillies, lemongrass, ginger, kaffir lime leaves and galangal, if using, then turn the heat down and simmer for 2 minutes.

Add the sugar, spring onions, prawns, fish sauce, tamari and lime juice, then return to the boil for 2–3 minutes until the prawns are cooked. Taste and adjust the seasoning, then add the mushrooms and heat through. At the last minute, add the coriander leaves and serve.

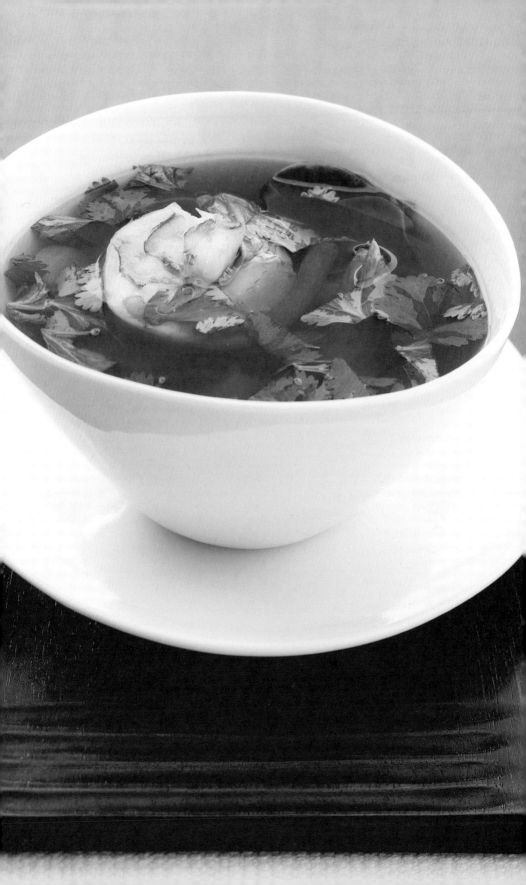

MAIN MEALS

The following meals are designed to provide plenty of nutrients to support brain health while minimizing blood-sugar spikes. Rich in protein, healthy fats and slow-release carbohydrates, they are quick and easy to assemble and many are suitable for freezing. You can serve these main meals with the suggested accompaniment or browse through the recipes for salads and side dishes on pages 159–165.

FRITTATA *[right]*

Serves 4

This is a versatile, dish that is equally delicious served cold in a packed lunch. Eggs are a great source of protein and choline, a key component of brain cell membranes.

150g (5½oz) new potatoes, peeled and
  quartered
1 tbsp coconut oil
1 red onion, finely sliced
2 courgettes, finely sliced
sprig of thyme, leaves scraped from
  the stalks
sea salt and freshly ground black
  pepper
6 eggs, beaten

Boil the potatoes until tender.
   Heat the oil in a large frying pan and soften the onion for 2–3 minutes over a very low heat without allowing it to brown. Add the courgettes, thyme leaves and a pinch of salt and freshly ground black pepper. Cook for another 3 minutes. Stir in the cooked potatoes and remove the pan from the heat.

Preheat the grill to medium. Pour the eggs into the pan with the vegetables and return it to the stove. Cook over a very low heat for about 8 minutes until the eggs are nearly set. Place the pan under the grill and cook until the eggs are completely set. Cut the frittata into generous wedges. Serve warm, or cold accompanied with a mixed leafy salad or Tomato and Wild Garlic Salad (*see* page 165).

STUFFED VEGETABLES

Serves 4

This makes a satisfying evening meal. Turkey is a rich source of the amino acid tryptophan, which serves as a precursor for serotonin, the neurotransmitter that helps the body regulate appetite, sleep patterns and mood. Vegetarians should replace the turkey with a little extra Mozzarella and a handful of walnuts.

2 large aubergines
1 tbsp coconut oil
1 onion, chopped
1 celery stick, chopped

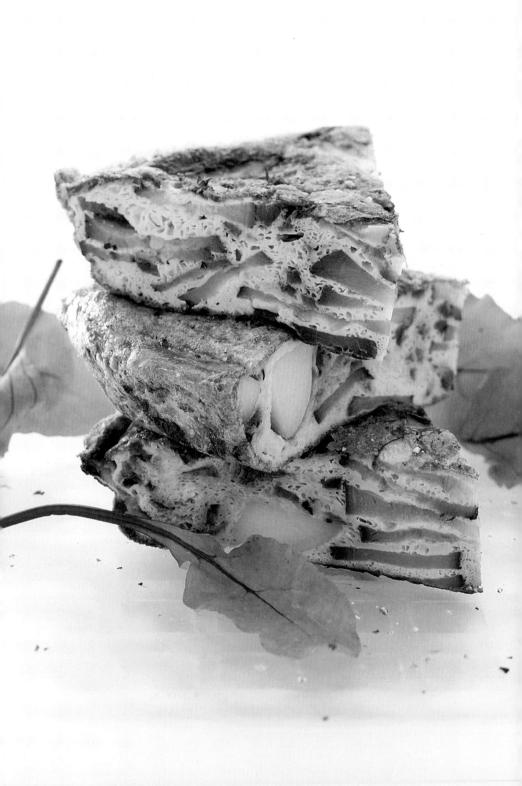

250g (9oz) turkey mince

50g (1¾oz/heaped ¼ cup) cooked
   mixed brown and wild rice

1 garlic clove, crushed

1 large tomato, peeled and chopped

50g (1¾oz) Mozzarella cheese, grated

Preheat the oven to 180°C (350°F/gas 4).
Slice the aubergines lengthways. Scoop
out the flesh, leaving about 1cm (½in) of
flesh inside the skin. Set the skins aside
and finely chop the aubergine flesh.

Heat the oil in a pan and soften the
aubergine flesh, onion and celery for 2
minutes. Add the turkey and stir-fry for
5 minutes until brown. Add the cooked
rice, garlic and tomato and stir well to
combine, then mix in half the cheese.
Fill the empty aubergine skins with the
mixture, top with the remaining cheese
and bake in the oven for 1 hour.

TURMERIC AND TAMARIND GLAZED SALMON

Serves 4

The marinade in this dish is rich in
the anti-inflammatory spice turmeric.
It would work well with other omega
3-rich fish such as mackerel or sardines.

3 tbsp ready-made tamarind paste

1 tbsp grated root ginger

2 garlic cloves, crushed

1 tsp sea salt

1 tsp turmeric

1 tbsp honey

4 boneless salmon fillets, skin on

1 tbsp coconut oil

Mix the tamarind paste, ginger, garlic,
salt, turmeric and honey together in a
large bowl until well combined.

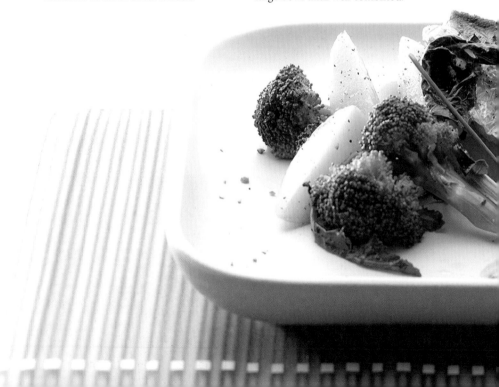

Add the salmon and mix well until completely coated. Cover and marinate for at least 1 hour, or place in the fridge and marinate overnight.

Heat the oil in a frying pan, add the salmon fillets and marinade and cook the salmon for 2–3 minutes on each side, basting occasionally with the marinade.

GRILLED RAINBOW TROUT [below]

Serves 4

This is a simple after-work supper dish. You could replace the trout with salmon fillets. Both are a useful source of omega 3 essential fats.

4 rainbow trout fillets, washed and dried
200ml (7fl oz/scant 1 cup) low-fat crème fraîche
100g (3½oz) cooked and peeled prawns
1 bunch of chives
lemon wedges, to serve

Place the fish fillets on a greased baking sheet and cook under a preheated grill for 2–3 minutes on each side. Meanwhile, in a saucepan, gently heat the crème fraîche with the prawns and chives. Pour the sauce over the fish to serve and accompany with lemon wedges and a Supergreens Salad (*see* page 161), or boiled new potatoes and steamed broccoli.

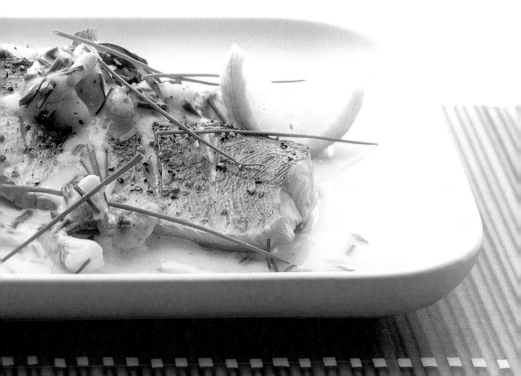

GRILLED HALIBUT WITH CARAMELIZED ONIONS

Serves 4

Halibut is a highly nutritious fish. It is rich in protein with a variety of important nutrients, including the minerals selenium, magnesium, phosphorus and potassium, plus the B vitamins B12, niacin, and B6, as well as omega 3 essential fatty acids.

zest and juice of 2 lemons
4 tbsp olive oil, plus extra for greasing
sea salt and freshly ground black
    pepper
4 boneless halibut fillets, skin on
4 onions, thinly sliced
1 tbsp chopped rosemary
1 tbsp chopped thyme
2 x 400-g (14-oz) tins plum tomatoes
4 tbsp balsamic vinegar
2 tbsp honey
1 handful of chopped parsley

Mix together the lemon zest and juice and 2 tablespoons of the oil. Season well, then pour over the halibut and leave to marinate for 30 minutes.

Heat the remaining oil in a pan and sauté the onions and herbs over a low heat for 10–15 minutes. Add the remaining ingredients and bubble for a further 20 minutes until the mixture has thickened.

Preheat the grill to high, place the fish on a greased baking sheet and cook under the grill for 2–3 minutes on each side until lightly golden and cooked through. Serve with the caramelized onion sauce.

THAI-SCENTED SEA BASS

Serves 4

Sea bass is an excellent source of protein and essential omega 3 fats important for balancing blood sugar and supporting brain-cell health. This delicious dish is simple to prepare and works well with other firm white fish

2.5cm (1in) piece of root ginger, peeled
    and grated
2 garlic cloves, crushed
zest and juice of 1 lime
2 tbsp tamari soy sauce
2 tbsp mirin
4 sea bass fillets, skin on

Place the ginger, garlic and lime zest and juice into an ovenproof baking dish. Add the tamari and mirin and stir well.

Place the sea bass in the baking dish and coat with the marinade. Cover and marinate for a couple of hours, if possible. Heat the oven to 200°C (400°F/ gas 6). Bake the fish for 20 minutes, or until the fish is cooked through. Serve with steamed or stir-fried vegetables and brown rice or Roasted Sweet Vegetables (*see* page 165).

TROUT WITH SUNFLOWER SEEDS

Serves 4

Sunflower seeds are an excellent source of vitamin E, a key fat-soluble antioxidant that is important for the protection of fat-containing cell membranes and brain cells.

4 whole trout, gutted and rinsed
  (head left on if wished)
juice of 2 lemons
1 tbsp olive oil
3 tbsp sunflower seeds

Preheat the oven to 200°C (400°F/ gas 6). Lay the fish in an ovenproof baking dish. Pour over the lemon juice and drizzle with the oil. Bake for 20 minutes, turning the trout halfway through the cooking time.

Toss the sunflower seeds in a dry frying pan over a medium heat until they are lightly toasted. Just before serving, sprinkle the seeds over the top of each trout.

GRILLED MACKEREL WITH CORIANDER PESTO

Serves 4

The tangy herb pesto works beautifully with the rich oily fish. Accompany with a mixed salad. Coriander is a fabulous cleansing herb packed with protective phytonutrients.

30g (1oz/scant ¼ cup) pine nuts
30g (1oz/scant ¼ cup) unsalted
  peanuts (optional)
1 green chilli, deseeded
1 garlic clove
1 large handful of coriander
1 tbsp tamari soy sauce
zest and juice of 1 lemon
2 tbsp olive oil
4 mackerel, rinsed and gutted
  (head left on if wished)

For the pesto, put the pine nuts, peanuts (if using), chilli, garlic, coriander and tamari in a food processor and purée until smooth. Add the lemon zest and 1 tablespoon lemon juice and enough of the oil to form a thick paste.

Preheat the grill to medium. Set aside half the pesto mixture and spoon the remaining quantity into the cavity of each mackerel.

Place the fish on a baking sheet and drizzle over a little extra lemon juice. Grill the fish for 5–6 minutes until cooked through. Serve with the reserved pesto and a mixed salad.

SALMON ROLLS *[page 148]*

Serves 4

These rice paper wraps are packed with protein but low in carbohydrates, making them an incredibly energizing dish. In place of rice paper sheets you could use large lettuce leaves instead.

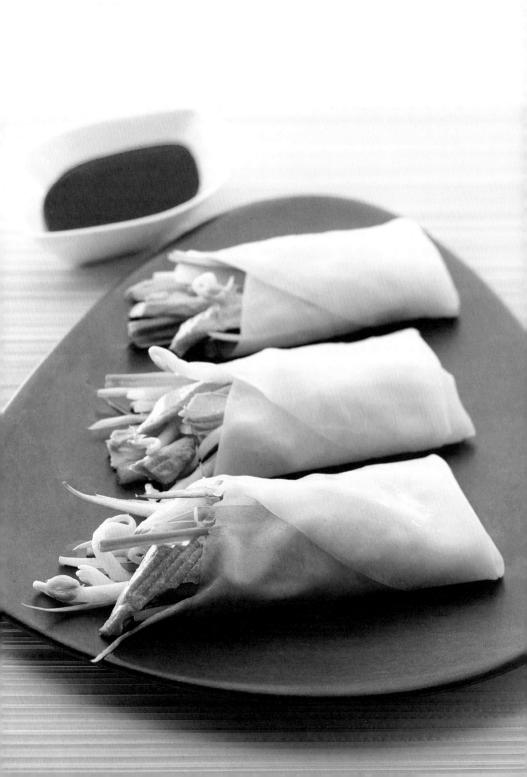

4 skinless, boneless salmon fillets
1 cucumber, sliced into long strips
4–6 spring onions, sliced
1 large handful of bean sprouts
125ml (4fl oz/½ cup) tamari soy sauce
2.5cm (1in) piece of root ginger, peeled
    and grated
3 tbsp toasted sesame oil
at least 16 rice pancakes

Steam or poach the salmon. When it is cooked, roughly break it up with a fork and leave it to cool in a serving bowl. Arrange the cucumber, spring onions and bean sprouts on a serving plate.

Mix the tamari, ginger and sesame oil and divide between two small serving bowls. Prepare the pancakes according to the instructions on the packet. Allow people to roll some salmon and vegetables in a pancake (or large lettuce leaf if using) and dip the rolls into the sauce before eating.

SESAME STIR-FRY

Serves 4

This chicken-and-vegetable stir-fry can be accompanied with whole-grain rice if wished. For speed use a bag of prepared stir-fry vegetables. If you like you can use about 180g (6¼oz) prawns or beef in place of the chicken.

2 skinless chicken breasts, cut into
    thin strips

1 tbsp tamari soy sauce
2.5cm (1in) piece of root ginger, peeled
    and finely sliced
1 garlic clove, finely sliced
2 tbsp coconut oil
1 tsp Chinese five-spice powder
1 handful of sugar snap peas or
    mangetout
1 onion, chopped
1 red pepper, cut into strips
1 carrot, cut into thin strips
1 tbsp coriander leaves, finely chopped
2 tbsp sesame seeds

Place the chicken in a bowl along with the tamari, ginger and garlic and mix well to coat the chicken.

Heat a wok or frying pan and add 1 tablespoon of the oil. Add the chicken and marinade to the pan and stir-fry until the chicken is cooked through. Remove the chicken with a slotted spoon (leaving any liquid in the pan), and set aside.

Heat the remaining oil in the pan and add the Chinese five-spice powder and all the prepared vegetables. Toss quickly and add 2 tablespoons water to steam-fry. Stir well on a high heat for about 2 minutes. Then put the chicken back into the pan and cook until reheated all the way through, without letting the vegetables become soft. At the last minute, scatter the coriander and sesame seeds over the top and serve.

SWEET ROAST LAMB

Serves 4

This is an excellent high-protein meal packed with energizing B vitamins and the antioxidants zinc and selenium. Leftovers can be eaten cold with salad for lunch, or reheated the next day.

1 leg of lamb
3 garlic cloves, sliced lengthways, plus
  1 whole garlic bulb
4 tbsp tamari soy sauce
2 tsp coarse-grain mustard
2 tsp honey
several rosemary stalks
12–15 cherry tomatoes

Preheat the oven to 190°C (375°F/gas 5). Wash the lamb and trim off any excess fat. Make incisions into the meat with a sharp knife and push slices of garlic into the slits. For the sauce, mix the tamari, mustard and honey in a bowl and add 2 tablespoons boiling water.

Place the lamb in a roasting pan on top of some of the rosemary and pour the sauce all over it. Place the garlic bulb beside the lamb and arrange the cherry tomatoes around the leg (the tomatoes will gradually turn mushy, but they add to the flavour of the gravy). Top with the rest of the rosemary.

Roast in the oven, basting every 20 minutes. Allow a cooking time of 55 minutes per kilogram (25 minutes per pound).

Add 125ml (4fl oz/½ cup) boiling water to the bottom of the roasting pan halfway through cooking to make a rich gravy.

Serve with freshly steamed broccoli or other green vegetables and roasted sweet potatoes.

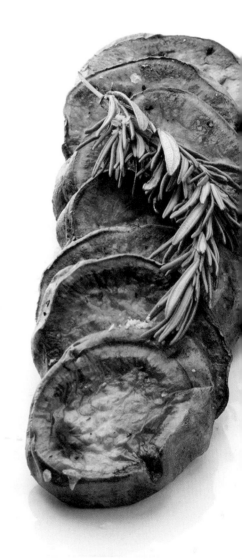

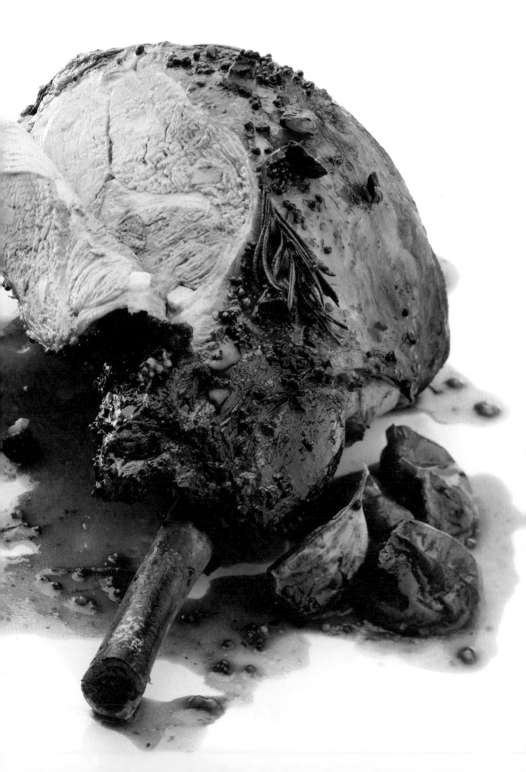

SEARED RASPBERRY DUCK

Serves 4

This delicious scented duck is equally delicious served cold in a packed lunch. A great source of protein, duck is also rich in niacin (B3), iron, selenium and calcium. Niacin helps to reduce low-density lipoprotein (LDL) cholesterol and helps to stabilize blood sugar by regulating the metabolism of insulin.

4 boneless duck breasts, skin on
sea salt and freshly ground black
**   pepper**
150g (5½oz) green beans, trimmed
250g (9oz) mixed green leaves
150g (5½oz) cherry tomatoes, halved
1 red onion, sliced

For the marinade:
4 tbsp tamari soy sauce
2 tbsp honey
6 tbsp raspberry vinegar
2 tbsp balsamic vinegar
4 tbsp olive oil
1 tsp Dijon mustard

Score the duck breasts on the fat side with a knife, season, and place in a shallow dish. Mix together all the marinade ingredients and pour over the duck breasts. Cover and leave to marinate for 1–2 hours, or overnight in the fridge.

Preheat the oven to 200°C (400°F/ gas 6). Heat an ovenproof frying pan, remove the duck breasts from the marinade, reserving the marinade, and sear them in the pan. Cook on a low heat for 10 minutes, then place the pan in the oven for a further 10 minutes.

Blanch the beans in boiling water for a couple of minutes then drain. Place the mixed leaves on a platter and top with the beans, tomatoes and onion. Allow the duck breasts to rest for 5 minutes then slice and place on top of the salad. Place the marinade in a pan and bring to the boil. Pour the sauce over the duck breasts to serve.

MACKEREL KEDGEREE

Serves 2

This is an omega 3-packed dish and is quick and easy to assemble. For a vegetarian option, omit the mackerel and use cooked tofu or hard-boiled eggs.

100g (3½oz/½ cup) brown rice
1 tbsp coconut oil
1 onion, finely diced
100g (3½oz) cherry tomatoes, halved
1 handful of sultanas
1 tsp turmeric
2 skinless smoked mackerel fillets
3 tbsp mixed seeds
2 tbsp chopped parsley

Cook the rice according to the packet instructions. About 10 minutes before the rice is cooked, heat the oil in a small pan and sauté the onion for 3–4 minutes until soft. Add the tomatoes, sultanas and turmeric and stir well. Break up the fish into large flakes. Drain the cooked rice and transfer to a large bowl. Add the contents of the pan and the flaked mackerel and mix well. Sprinkle over the seeds and parsley and serve with a leafy green salad.

CUMIN-SPICED STEAK WITH HERB SALSA

Serves 4

Grass-fed lean beef is rich in protein, healthy fats and homocysteine-lowering B vitamins, making it a healthy brain food. This easy dinner dish is simple to prepare and leftovers would make an ideal accompaniment to a salad for lunch the next day.

500g (1lb 2oz) boned beef fillet
sea salt and freshly ground black
pepper
1 tsp ground cumin
1 garlic clove, crushed
3 tbsp olive oil

For the salsa:
1 handful of coriander leaves, chopped
1 red onion, chopped
a pinch of cayenne pepper
1 red chilli, deseeded and finely
chopped

a pinch of sea salt
1 ripe mango, diced
juice of 1 lime

Place the beef fillet in a shallow bowl and season well. Mix together the cumin, garlic and oil and pour over the beef. Cover and leave to marinate for 1–2 hours, or overnight in the fridge if possible.

Preheat the oven to 200°C (400°F/ gas 6). Heat an ovenproof frying pan over a high heat and quickly brown the beef fillet on all sides, then place in the oven and roast for 15–20 minutes. Remove from the oven and leave to rest for 5 minutes.

Mix together all the ingredients for the salsa. Slice the beef into thin strips and serve with the salsa on the side and accompanied by a green salad.

SHIITAKE CHICKEN

Serves 4

This is a variation on the traditional roast. Shiitake mushrooms are known for supporting the immune system and are an excellent source of B vitamins, including B5 needed to support the adrenal glands in times of stress. Their nutty flavour helps create a rich gravy.

1.5kg (3lb 5oz) organic chicken
4 garlic cloves, sliced, plus 2–3 whole
garlic cloves

4 tbsp tamari soy sauce
1 lemon
8–12 dried shiitake mushrooms
freshly ground black pepper
2 tsp honey
250ml (9fl oz/1 cup) hot chicken stock
  or boiling water

Preheat the oven to 190°C (375°F/gas 5). Place the chicken in a roasting tin. Use a sharp knife to make incisions in the fleshy legs of the chicken and insert slices of garlic into the slits. Put the whole garlic cloves in the bottom of the roasting pan. Pour over the tamari and rub all over the bird. Cut the lemon in half and squeeze the juice all over the chicken. Then cut one of the squeezed lemon halves into three and place in the roasting tin. Place the other lemon half inside the cavity of the bird. Arrange the shiitake mushrooms around the chicken and grind black pepper all over it.

Dissolve the honey in the chicken stock or water and pour into the bottom of the roasting pan.

Roast the chicken in the oven for about 1¼ hours, or until the juices from the chicken run clear when the thickest part of the thigh is pierced with a sharp knife. Baste the meat every 20 minutes during cooking.

Serve with steamed greens and Roasted Sweet Vegetables (*see* page 165).

LENTILS WITH SPINACH
[right]
Serves 4

Lentils provide plenty of fibre and slow-release carbohydrates, helping to balance blood-sugar levels and keeping the body energized. They are also a great vegetarian source of iron. If time is short use a can of cooked lentils instead. For additional protein add chunks of feta cheese at the end of cooking.

250g (9oz/1⅓ cups) brown lentils
½ tsp ground coriander
½ tsp ground cumin
1 garlic clove, crushed
1 tbsp olive oil
sea salt and freshly ground black
  pepper
500g (1lb 2oz) fresh spinach, chopped

Put the lentils in a pan of cold water, bring to the boil and then simmer for about an hour until they are soft. Put the coriander, cumin, garlic and oil in a pan and season with salt and pepper. Stir for about a minute over a medium heat. Add the spinach and stir for a couple more minutes. Drain the lentils, combine with the spinach mixture in the pan and serve.

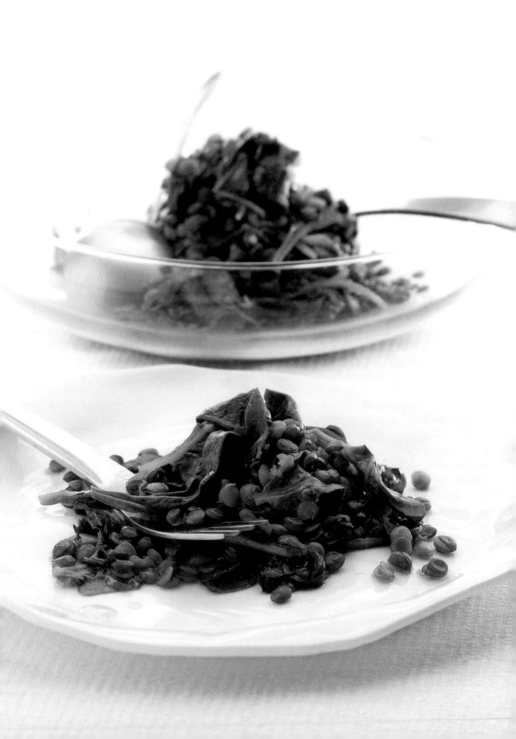

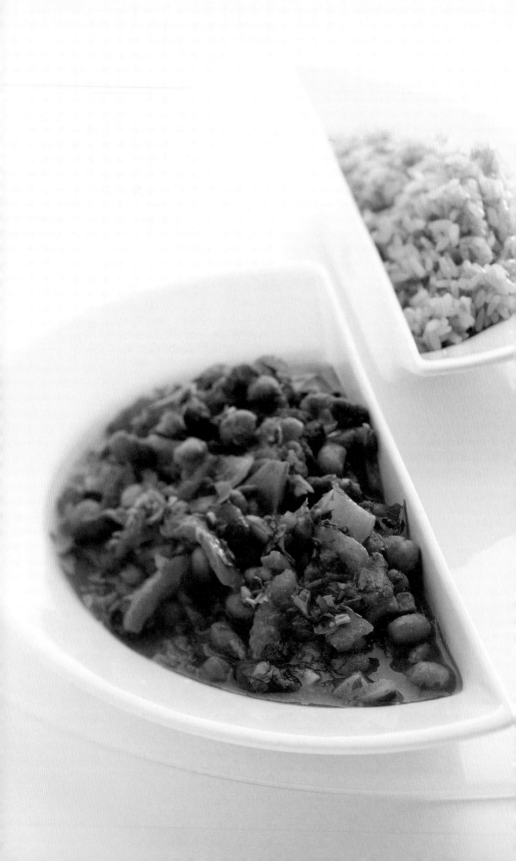

SPICED BEAN STEW *[left]*

Serves 3–4

This is a perfect warming, one-pot dish for the winter. It is lightly spiced and full of flavour. You could add chunks of sweet potato to make it more substantial if you wish.

1 tbsp coconut oil

1 onion, chopped

2 garlic cloves, crushed

1 tsp ground cumin

½ tsp cardamom

½ tsp paprika

½ tsp ground cinnamon

3 large tomatoes, peeled and
  chopped

2 x 420-g (15-oz) tins mixed beans,
  drained

1 handful of chopped parsley,
  to serve

Heat the oil in a frying pan and sauté the onion and garlic for 2 minutes. Add the spices and stir well for a few minutes. Add the tomatoes and beans. Pour in a little water if needed, cover, and simmer for 20 minutes. Serve the stew garnished with a generous amount of chopped parsley and accompanied by brown rice if wished.

GINGERED LAMB TAGINE

Serves 4

This Moroccan-style tagine is made wonderfully sweet with the addition of prunes. Prunes are a great source of protective phytonutrients and fibre important for lowering cholesterol. Serve with whole-grain rice and steamed vegetables.

500g (1lb 2oz) lamb steak, cut into
  chunks

plain flour, for coating

sea salt and freshly ground black
  pepper

coconut oil, for frying

2 onions, chopped

2 garlic cloves, crushed

1 carrot, sliced

2cm (¾in) piece of root ginger, peeled
  and grated

1 tsp ground cumin

1 tsp ground cinnamon

1 tsp ground coriander

300ml (10½fl oz/scant 1¼ cups)
  lamb stock

100ml (3½fl oz/generous ⅓ cup)
  red wine

1 tbsp honey

125g (4½oz) ready-to-eat prunes

1 handful of chopped coriander

Toss the lamb in the flour and season. Heat a tablespoon of the oil in a frying pan over a fairly high heat and brown the lamb on all sides. Remove from the pan. Add a little more oil to the pan and sauté the onions, garlic, carrot, ginger and spices for 2 minutes. Add the stock, wine, honey, prunes and meat and bring to the boil. Turn the heat down, cover, and simmer gently for 1 hour until the meat is very tender. Add the coriander at the last minute and serve.

QUINOA WITH ROAST VEGETABLES

Serves 4

Quinoa is a nutritious grain providing a complete source of protein and high levels of calcium, phosphorous, iron and B vitamins, including brain-boosting B6, B3, B1 and B2, plus vitamin E to protect the fatty membranes of brain cells.

1 red pepper, deseeded and cut into
   chunks
1 green pepper, deseeded and cut into
   chunks
2 red onions, quartered
2 courgettes, cut into chunks
2 large Portobello mushrooms, thickly
   sliced
8–10 cherry tomatoes
8–10 garlic cloves
olive oil, for roasting
a few thyme sprigs
sea salt and freshly ground black
   pepper
180g (6½oz/scant 1 cup) quinoa, rinsed
500ml (17fl oz/2 cups) vegetable stock

Preheat the oven to 180°C (350°F/gas 4).

Toss all the vegetables together with the garlic in a large roasting tin with plenty of oil and the thyme. Season with freshly ground black pepper and a little sea salt. Roast in the oven for 30–40 minutes, or until all the vegetables are tender and golden.

Place the quinoa in a pan with the stock. Bring to the boil, then turn the heat down, cover and simmer for 15 minutes. Remove from the heat and allow to stand for 5 minutes. Spoon the quinoa onto a platter and top with the roasted vegetables to serve.

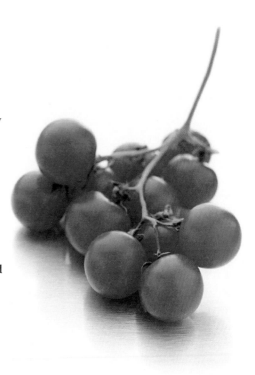

SIDE DISHES

CRUNCHY ORIENTAL SALAD

Serves 2–3

30g (1oz) dried sea vegetables, such
   as arame
2 carrots, grated
¼ red cabbage, shredded
3 spring onions, finely sliced
2 tbsp chopped coriander
Oriental Sesame Dressing, to serve
   (*see* page 159)
1 tbsp sesame seeds, to serve

Put the sea vegetables in a pan and
cover with boiling water. Allow to soak
for 10 minutes then drain.

   Put the carrots into a large bowl
with the cabbage, spring onions and
coriander. Scatter over the sea vegetable
then add the dressing and toss. Sprinkle
over the sesame seeds to serve.

SALAD DRESSINGS

Salad dressings are a great way to boost
your intake of healthy fats, which is why
many of the recipes below make use
of omega 3-rich oils such as flaxseed,
omega 3·6·9 balance oils, walnut oil and
hemp seed oil.

   For all of these dressings, simply place
the ingredients into a screw-top jar and
shake well. They will keep in the fridge
for at least a week.

CREAMY VINAIGRETTE

3 tbsp extra-virgin olive oil
3 tbsp flaxseed oil
2 tbsp balsamic vinegar
1 heaped tsp coarse-grain mustard
freshly ground black pepper

SWEET AND TANGY VINAIGRETTE

1 tbsp sherry vinegar
1 tbsp balsamic vinegar
3 tbsp extra-virgin olive oil
1 tbsp hemp seed oil
2 tbsp flaxseed oil
1 tsp Dijon mustard
1 garlic clove, crushed
a pinch of dried red chilli flakes
sea salt and freshly ground black
   pepper

ORIENTAL SESAME DRESSING

2 tbsp omega 3·6·9 oil
2 tsp sesame oil
juice of 2 limes
3 tbsp tamari soy sauce
1 tbsp rice vinegar
2 tbsp honey
1 tsp grated root ginger
1 garlic clove, crushed

RICH PESTO DRESSING

2 tsp ready-made pesto
4 tbsp omega 3·6·9 oil
2 tbsp lemon juice
freshly ground black pepper

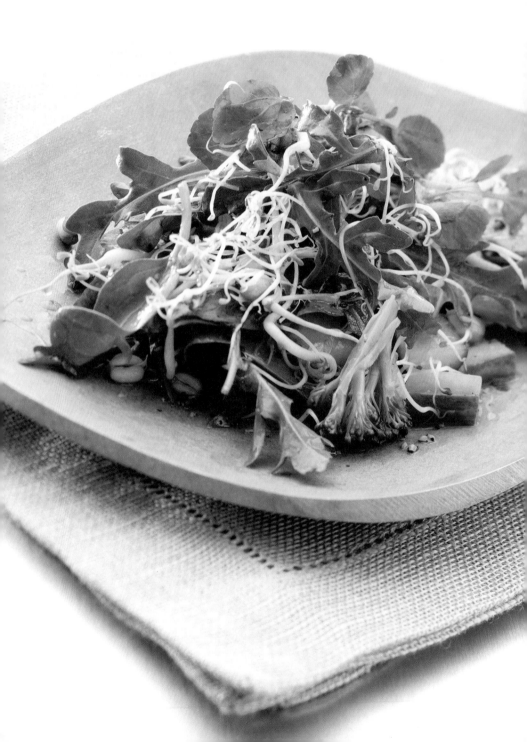

SUPERGREENS SALAD

[left]

Serves 2–4

This salad is packed with leafy greens
and vegetables, providing a wealth of
nutrients and healthy fats. Serve this
as a main salad, if wished, accompanied
with some protein such as grilled
chicken or prawns.

2 handfuls of baby spinach
4 broccoli florets, trimmed and lightly
    steamed if wished
2 tbsp shredded white cabbage
1 handful of watercress
1 handful of rocket
1 handful of sprouted alfalfa
1 handful of sprouted mung beans
5cm (2in) cucumber, diced
1 ripe avocado, peeled, pitted and
    diced
1 tbsp pumpkin seeds

Toss all the ingredients together in a
large bowl and serve with one of the
salad dressings on page 159.

GREEN PAPAYA SALAD

Serves 4

Green papaya, popular in Asian dishes,
is an unripe large papaya that soaks up
the delicious flavours of the dressing.
This side dish is light and refreshing
and makes an ideal accompaniment
to prawns or Thai spiced fish.

1 green papaya, peeled and finely
    shredded
4 spring onions, thinly sliced
200g (7oz) cherry tomatoes,
    halved
1 cucumber, deseeded and cut into
    julienne strips
1 handful of basil leaves, chopped
1 handful of mint leaves, chopped
1 handful of coriander leaves, chopped
2 tbsp roasted cashew nuts

For the dressing:
juice of 2 limes
1 tsp sugar
½ red chilli, deseeded and chopped
1 tbsp fish sauce
1 garlic clove, crushed

Mix together the ingredients for the
dressing and set aside.

Place all the other ingredients in a
large bowl and mix together. Drizzle
over the dressing and toss before
serving.

QUINOA TABBOULEH *[below]*

Serves 2–3

This delicious Middle Eastern salad is made using quinoa, which is gluten-free, rather than traditional bulgar wheat. Use plenty of parsley to really lift the flavour of this dish. It is perfect with meat or fish as a side dish, or serve as a vegetarian main course with some additional protein such as feta cheese or hard-boiled eggs.

180g (6¼oz/scant 1 cup) quinoa
500ml (17fl oz/2 cups) vegetable stock
a pinch of saffron
large bunch of parsley, finely chopped
1 large handful of mint, finely chopped
6 spring onions, finely sliced

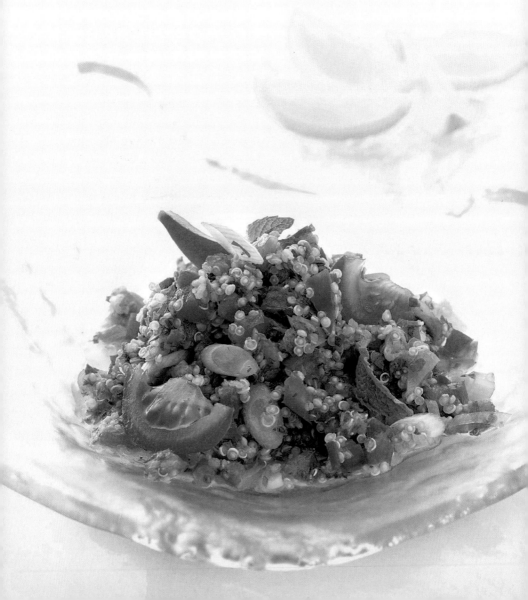

1 tsp ground cumin

½ cucumber, deseeded and finely chopped

4 vine-ripe tomatoes, roughly chopped

2 tbsp flaxseed oil

2 tbsp olive oil

zest and juice of 1 lemon

sea salt and freshly ground black pepper

Place the quinoa in a pan with the vegetable stock and saffron. Bring to the boil, then turn the heat down, cover and simmer gently for 15 minutes. Remove from the heat and allow to stand for 5 minutes, then fluff up with a fork. Place in a large bowl and mix in the remaining ingredients. Season to taste.

FENNEL AND CARROT SALAD [below]

Serves 2

A simple but delicious side salad. Fennel is a well-known digestive aid and is rich in phytonutrients shown to reduce inflammation. This is best served as an accompaniment to meat or fish dishes.

3 carrots, grated

1 fennel bulb, cored and finely sliced

3 spring onions, finely sliced

juice of 1 orange

2 tbsp olive oil

1 tbsp toasted sunflower seeds

Toss the carrots together with the fennel, spring onions, orange juice and oil. Scatter the sunflower seeds over and serve with lemon wedges, if wished.

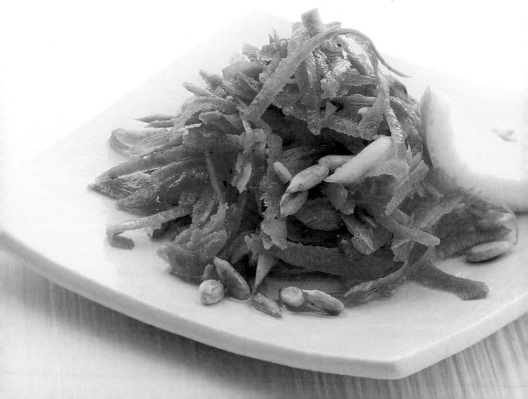

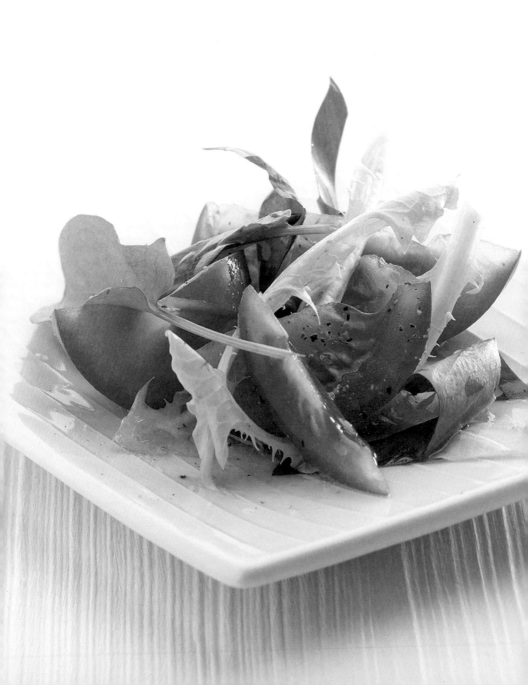

TOMATO AND WILD GARLIC SALAD *[left]*

Serves 2

Light and refreshing, choose vine-ripe tomatoes for this salad recipe for maximum flavour.

1 handful of sorrel or rocket leaves
1 handful of wild garlic stalks or chives, chopped
2 vine-ripe tomatoes, cut into quarters
shavings of Parmesan (optional)
2 tbsp extra-virgin olive oil
2 tbsp lemon juice
sea salt and freshly ground black pepper

Toss the sorrel leaves, wild garlic, tomatoes and Parmesan (if using) in a bowl and drizzle with the oil and lemon juice. Season to taste.

ROASTED SWEET VEGETABLES

Serves 4

Creamy butternut squash roasted with earthy beetroot and drizzled with a spicy dressing makes the base for a warming winter salad or accompaniment to meat and fish dishes. Turn this into a vegetarian main meal by adding some goat's cheese and toasted pine nuts.

1 large sweet potato, peeled and cut into chunks
1 butternut squash, peeled and cut into cubes
2 beetroot, peeled and cut into chunks
1 garlic clove, crushed
2 tbsp red wine vinegar
1 tbsp honey
4 tbsp olive oil
a pinch of dried red chilli flakes

Preheat the oven to 190°C (375°F/gas 5). Place the sweet potato, butternut squash and beetroots on a baking tray. Mix together the garlic, red wine vinegar, honey, oil and chilli flakes and drizzle half of the mixture over the vegetables. Toss to coat. Bake the vegetables in the oven for 20–30 minutes until tender. Drizzle over the remaining dressing before serving.

DESSERTS

In this section you will find a range of low-sugar recipes for desserts as well as baked treats – perfect for packed lunches. None contain refined sugar and all are carefully balanced to help stabilize blood sugar. The focus is on providing the body with nutritious ingredients to boost your energy levels, and balance blood glucose essential for optimum brain health and function.

APRICOT ICE CREAM WITH PISTACHIOS [right]

Serves 4

Using dried apricots provides natural sweetness without the need to add extra sugar. The chopped pistachio nuts provide a wonderful nutty crunch to this ice cream as well as additional protein.

100g (3½oz) dried apricots, soaked
    overnight in water and drained
150ml (5fl oz/scant ⅔ cup) plain
    Greek yogurt
½ tsp ground cardamom
60g (2¼oz/scant ½ cup) shelled
    pistachio nuts, crushed, plus extra

Blend the apricots with the yogurt and cardamom in a food processor. Fold the pistachios into the apricot mixture.

Pour the mixture into a freezable container and freeze for 2–3 hours, or until firm. Stir every 40 minutes to prevent ice crystals from forming.

If you freeze the ice cream for longer than 3 hours, put it in the fridge for 20 minutes before serving. Serve topped with a extra chopped pistachios.

SPICED FRUITS

Serves 4

500ml (17fl oz/2 cups) apple juice
15 cardamom pods, split
1 cinnamon stick
2 star anise
100g (3½oz) dried pears
100g (3½oz) dried peaches
100g (3½oz) dried apricots

For the vanilla yogurt:
300ml (10½fl oz/scant 1¼ cups) plain
    Greek yogurt
2 tsp vanilla extract

Place the apple juice in a pan with the spices, heat gently and simmer for 5 minutes. Add the dried fruits and simmer over a low heat for 10 minutes. In a separate bowl, mix the yogurt with the vanilla extract. Serve the fruit hot or cold with the vanilla yogurt.

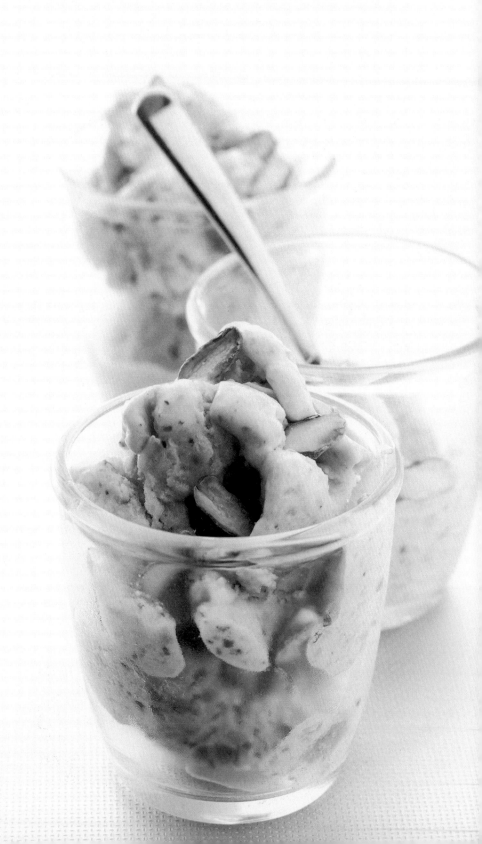

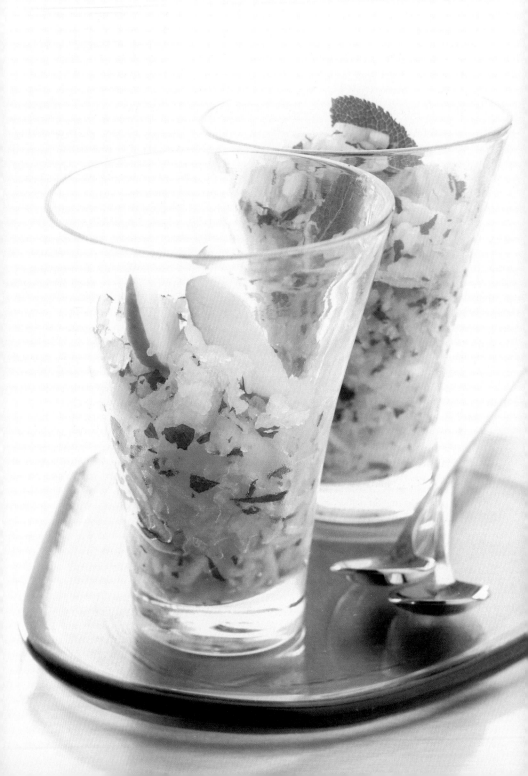

CHOCOLATE PUDDING

Serves 4

Rich and indulgent-tasting yet low in sugar, this is perfect for special occasions. You can make this a dairy-free dessert by using a milk alternative and dairy-free chocolate.

600ml (21fl oz/scant 2½ cups) semi-skimmed milk or milk alternative
75–100g (2½–3½oz) dark, organic chocolate
4 eggs
¼ tsp sea salt
1 tsp vanilla extract

Preheat the oven to 170°C (325°F/ gas 3). Put the milk and chocolate in a saucepan over a low heat, stirring gently until the chocolate is melted and well mixed in with the milk. Do not allow it to boil. Remove from the heat and leave to cool.

Put the eggs, salt and vanilla extract in a blender, slowly add the chocolate milk and blend until well mixed. Pour into 4 ramekin dishes. Place the ramekins on a baking tray and bake in the oven for 40 minutes.

Serve hot or allow to cool and chill, covered with a little cling film, until ready to serve.

GRATED APPLE ICE *[left]*

Serves 4

This makes a refreshing light dessert. The pectin from the apples and the addition of mint are useful for supporting digestive health.

4 Granny Smith apples (or another sharp variety)
1 tbsp lemon juice
2 tbsp Manuka honey
2 tbsp rose- or orange-blossom water
4 ice cubes
4 mint sprigs, leaves torn

Retain 4 thin slices of apple for the garnish. Peel and grate the rest of the apples into a glass bowl. Pour the lemon juice over them and stir well. Add the honey and rose-water and stir again. Chill for at least 2 hours.

Before serving, crush the ice cubes in a blender or mortar and pestle and add to the apple mix. Stir the mint leaves into the apple ice. Serve garnished with the slices of apple.

CHOCOLATE BANANA MOUSSE

Serves 2

Adding avocado to this pudding creates a wonderfully rich dessert packed with healthy fats and plenty of antioxidant vitamin E. Raw cacao powder is high in protective antioxidants while the cashew nut butter adds protein and healthy fats. For additional protein you could add a scoop of chocolate or vanilla protein powder.

2 ripe bananas
1 ripe avocado, peeled and pitted
1 tbsp melted coconut oil
4 tbsp raw cacao powder
1 tbsp Manuka honey
1 tbsp cashew nut butter
1 scoop chocolate or vanilla protein
   powder (optional)
coconut flakes and cacao nibs, to
   garnish

Place the bananas, avocado, oil, cacao powder, honey, nut butter and protein powder (if using) in a blender and process until smooth and creamy. Spoon into glasses and top with a few coconut flakes and cacao nibs to serve.

WALNUT OAT CRUMBLE

Serves 4

The addition of nuts in the crumble mix provides protein and healthy fats. Bags of frozen berries are perfect for making instant puddings especially when fresh berries are out of season.

150g (5½oz/1½ cups) walnuts
250g (9oz) no-added-sugar muesli
2 tsp ground cinnamon
3 tbsp melted coconut oil
4 tbsp apple juice
500g (1lb 2oz) fresh or frozen mixed
   berries
1 tbsp arrowroot

Preheat the oven to 190°C (350°F/gas 5). Place the walnuts in a blender and process to form fine crumbs. Put the walnuts, muesli and cinnamon into a large bowl, pour over the coconut oil and apple juice and mix well.

Place the berries in a baking dish and sprinkle over the arrowroot and 2 tablespoons water. Mix lightly. Spread the crumble mix over the berries and bake in the oven for 30 minutes until the top is golden brown. Serve with vanilla yogurt (*see* page 166).

LEMON COCONUT BARS

Makes 12–16 bars

An iced dessert sweetened with dates and xylitol rather than refined sugar. Adding lecithin provides an additional source of choline – an important nutrient for protecting brain function and memory.

250g (9oz/1⅔ cups) almonds
150g (5½oz/1⅔ cups) desiccated
   coconut
400g (14oz/2¼ cups) soft pitted dates,
   such as Medjool or Khadrawi
zest and juice of 1 lemon
2 tsp vanilla extract

For the topping:
250g (9oz/1⅔ cups) cashews, soaked
   in water for 2 hours
300ml (10½fl oz/1¼ cups) coconut milk
zest and juice of 2 lemons
60g (2¼oz) xylitol
1 tbsp vanilla extract
1 tsp turmeric
125ml (4fl oz/½ cup) coconut oil
2 tbsp lecithin powder

Place the almonds in a food processor and process until very fine. Add the coconut, dates, lemon zest and juice and vanilla and process until combined. Press the mixture into a lined baking tray, about 20–22cm (8–8½in) square.

Place all the filling ingredients except the oil and lecithin powder in a high-speed blender and process until thick and creamy. Add the oil and lecithin and process quickly to combine. Pour over the base and spread evenly. Place in the freezer and chill for 1–2 hours until firm. Cut into bars to serve.

MACA ICE CREAM

Serves 4

Maca is a delicious superfood known for its ability to help the body cope with stress. This dairy-free ice cream is simple to prepare, high in protein and low in sugar.

280g (10oz/1¾ cups) cashews
2–3 tbsp Manuka honey to taste
1 vanilla pod, split in half and seeds
   scraped out (discard the pod)
700ml (24fl oz/2¾ cups) almond milk
   or coconut milk
3 tbsp maca root powder
1 tsp lemon juice
a pinch of sea salt

Place all the ingredients in a high-speed blender and process until smooth. Pour into an ice-cream maker and churn according to the manufacturer's instructions.

Alternatively, pour into a freezable container and place in the freezer for 2 hours. Remove from the freezer and beat in a food processor until smooth. Return to the freezer until required.

GINGERED PEARS *[right]*

Serves 4

A warming fruit dessert that is delicious hot or cold. This would also make a wonderful breakfast option served with some mixed seeds.

2 tbsp Manuka honey

1.25cm (½in) piece of root ginger, peeled and finely sliced

2 tbsp kirsch

4 firm pears, peeled and halved lengthways

6 tbsp crème fraîche

½ tsp ground cinnamon

4 mint leaves, to garnish (optional)

Preheat the oven to 180°C (350°F/gas 4). Put the honey, ginger and 500ml (17fl oz/2 cups) water in a saucepan and bring to the boil. Lower the heat and simmer for 10 minutes. Add the kirsch. Meanwhile, lay the pears in an ovenproof dish.

Pour the ginger sauce over the pears and bake in the oven for 30 minutes until soft.

Mix the crème fraîche with the cinnamon. Place two pear halves in each bowl and put a dollop of the cinnamon crème fraîche on top. Garnish with a mint leaf if wished.

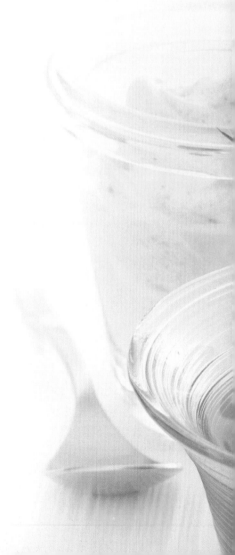

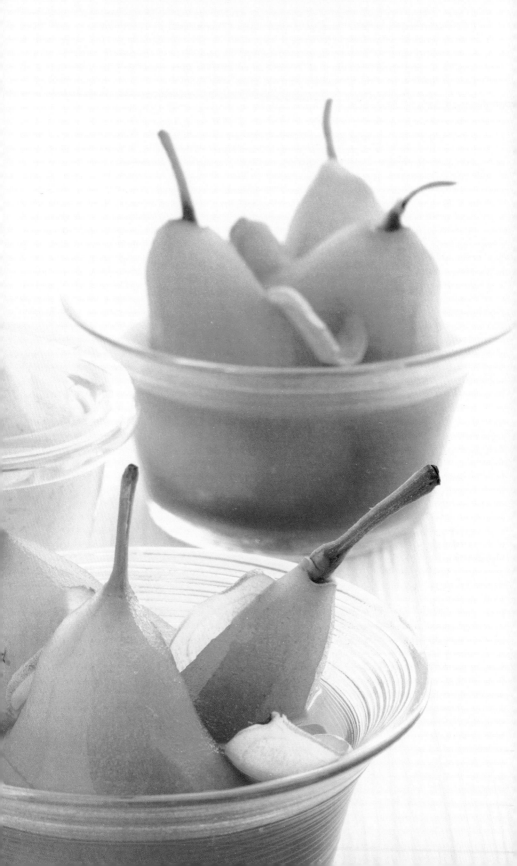

SNACKS

Including a healthy snack between meals is a useful way to balance blood-sugar levels to keep yourself feeling energized and focused throughout the day. To avoid energy dips choose snacks that combine a slow-releasing carbohydrate with some healthy fat and protein. Here are some simple ideas.

FRESH FRUIT WITH NATURAL YOGURT
Choose low-glycaemic load fruit such as citrus fruits, berries, apples, pears, plums and apricots. Top with natural yogurt and a tablespoon of mixed seeds.

FRESH NUTS AND SEEDS
Go for fresh almonds, hazelnuts, cashews or Brazils, and avoid nuts that are roasted or salted. For seeds, have a mixture of pumpkin, sunflower and sesame. Chew them all well to get the most out of their goodness. These are easily portable and make a healthy snack on the go.

VEGETABLE STICKS WITH MEAT AND/OR FISH
Cut up a range of raw vegetables ready for snacking on. Accompany with slices of cooked lean meats, ham, fish or prawns or choose a dip such as guacamole, hummus or cottage cheese.

CRACKERS WITH TOPPINGS
Choose from oatcakes, whole-grain rice cakes or rye crackers and top them with:
* hummus, goat's cheese or cottage cheese with tomatoes
* nut and seed butters (unsalted and unsweetened)
* Mackerel Pâté (*see* page 126)

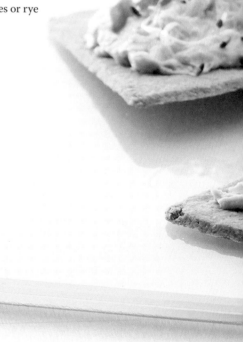

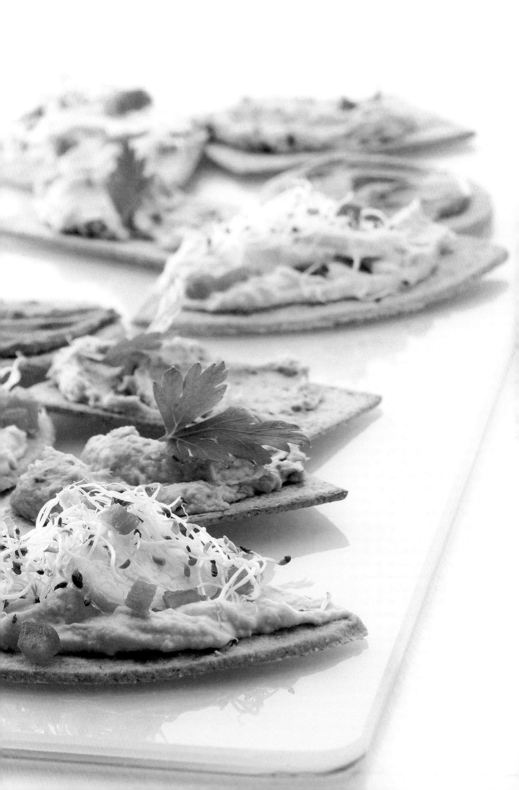

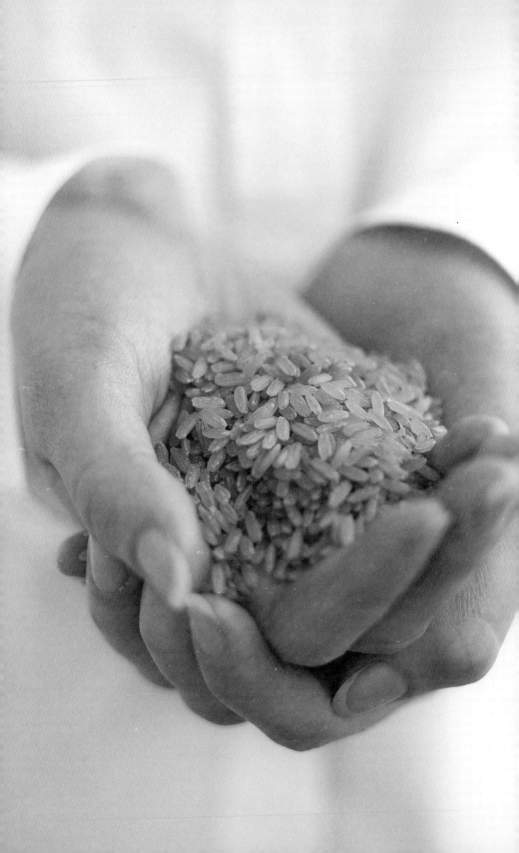

THE WHOLE
PICTURE

Good nutrition forms just one part of the mind–body canvas, and dietary improvements alone are not always enough to overcome ongoing low moods. In this chapter we explore a range of strategies to complement a balanced diet and help to keep you in peak physical and emotional health.

As well as eating a good diet based on the advice given in the first three chapters, you could consider taking nutritional supplements – these optimize your nutritional status and can dramatically enhance how you feel. However, to complete the picture of good health and to maintain even moods, it is also essential that you make other positive lifestyle changes. Doing regular, gentle exercise, sharing your problems and inner feelings with someone else (whether that person is a friend or a professional), and being aware of your approach to major life events can provide you with the sense of equilibrium that is essential for a joyful, fulfilling existence.

FEEL-GOOD SUPPLEMENTS

Taking nutritional supplements that are right for you can boost your energy and mood, minimize your risk of getting ill and generally help you look and feel better. However, supplements should not replace a healthy, balanced diet, and are best taken with professional guidance.

Positive as nutritional supplements can be, we must not forget what they are. It may seem obvious but, as their name suggests, they are meant to supplement a good diet – they are not a substitute for one. It's all too easy to cut corners with our diets, mistakenly hoping for a quick fix from popping pills. Unfortunately, feeling good doesn't come as simply or mechanically as that.

Whether we actually need to take supplements at all is a subject of much debate. Traditionalists may argue that we can get all the nutrients we need from a good diet. Indeed, a varied, balanced, healthy diet consisting of chemical-free, fresh food and void of substances that drain nutrients, such as alcohol and fizzy, sweet drinks, would probably provide an optimum nutrient intake. However, very few of us manage consistently to eat that well. Some of the opponents of food supplements may claim that there has been too little research into their use, particularly at high doses. In some cases this may be a valid argument, although a great deal more scientific research has been done into the benefits and safety of natural nutrients than many may realize.

If you do choose to take supplements, deciding which are best for you can in itself be a minefield. Your local health shop or pharmacy probably stocks countless supplements, each claiming purported benefits and a wide range of qualities. Although we all have different individual nutritional requirements, a basic programme can make a great difference to how you feel. The best place to start is with a good, all-round, multi-supplement to cover all bases: one that contains all the vitamins, most minerals and perhaps even a few extras, such as plant extracts with antioxidant or cleansing properties. When choosing a multi-supplement, bear in mind that, as with most things in life, you usually get what you pay for, so cutting costs can sometimes be a false economy. Other than basic multi-supplements, any food supplements are best taken under the guidance of a qualified nutritionist or other health professional. If you are pregnant or on medication, it is essential that you seek advice from your doctor.

Controversy also surrounds the issue of supplement dosage. There are often large discrepancies between governments' recommended daily intakes and those recommended by some health practitioners. This gap is, in part, owing to the fact that most standard state recommendations are based on the amount of a nutrient required to

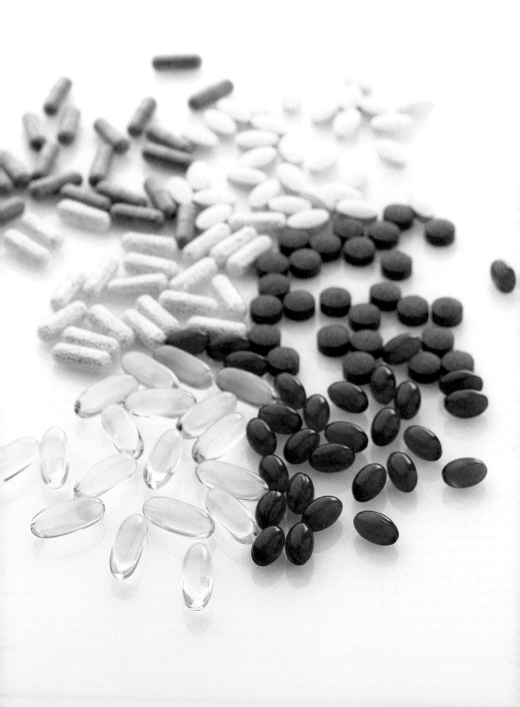

prevent symptoms of a deficiency. However, research and practice usually show that much higher levels are required for optimum health. As long as you follow the recommendations given by your health practitioner or printed on the bottle of a supplement, you are unlikely to experience any adverse effects.

The ideal is to have a personal supplements programme designed by a qualified nutritionist. Nevertheless, you can make a tremendous difference by following the general recommendations in this book, even without your own tailored programme. Just remember to use the supplements to *support* a diet rich in vitamins and minerals. See the next few pages for a list of the most essential nutrients and their rich food sources.

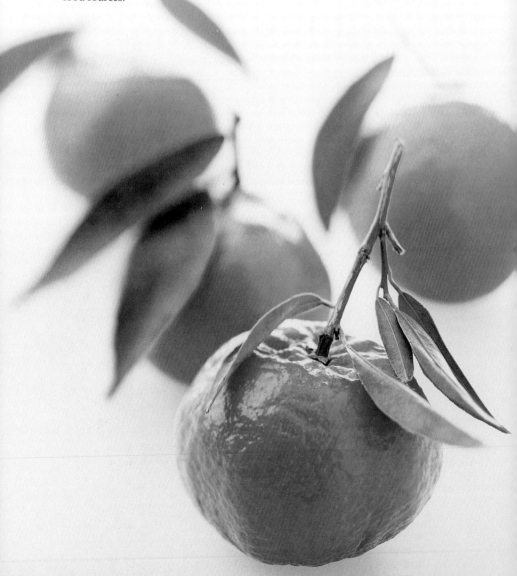

NUTRIENTS AND THEIR RICH FOOD SOURCES

NUTRIENT	RICH FOOD SOURCES
Vitamin A/ Beta-carotene	Apricots, asparagus, broccoli, cantaloupe melon, carrots, kale, liver, pumpkin, spinach, sweet potatoes, watermelon
Vitamin D (cholecalciferol)	Cod liver oil, herring, mackerel, salmon, sardines
Vitamin E (alpha tocopherol)	Almonds, avocado, corn oil, hazelnuts, sunflower seeds and oil, walnuts, wheatgerm, whole-grain flour
Vitamin C (ascorbic acid)	Blackcurrants, broccoli, Brussels sprouts, cabbage, grapefruit, guava, kale, lemons, oranges, papaya, peppers, potatoes, spinach, strawberries, tomatoes, watercress
Vitamin B1 (thiamine)	Beef kidney and liver, brewer's yeast, brown rice, chickpeas, kidney beans, pork, rice bran, salmon, soya beans, sunflower seeds, wheatgerm, whole-grain wheat and rye
Vitamin B2 (riboflavin)	Almonds, brewer's yeast, cheese, chicken, mushrooms, wheatgerm
Vitamin B3 (niacin)	Beef liver, brewer's yeast, chicken, eggs, fish, sunflower seeds, turkey
Vitamin B5 (pantothenic acid)	Blue cheese, brewer's yeast, carrots, corn, eggs, lentils, liver, lobster, meats, peanuts, peas, soya beans, sunflower seeds, wheatgerm, whole-grain products
Vitamin B6 (pyridoxine)	Avocados, bananas, bran, brewer's yeast, carrots, hazelnuts, lentils, rice, salmon, shrimps, soya beans, sunflower seeds, tuna, walnuts, wheatgerm, whole-grain flour

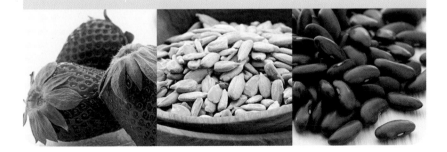

NUTRIENTS AND THEIR RICH FOOD SOURCES

NUTRIENT	RICH FOOD SOURCES
Vitamin B12 (cyanocobalamin)	Cheese, clams, eggs, fish, meat, milk and milk products
Antioxidants	Avocados, beetroot, berries, broccoli, cabbage, carrots, figs, fish, garlic, grapes, green tea, kale, nuts, onions, peppers, prunes, raisins, seeds, sweet potatoes, tomatoes, watercress, wheatgerm
Biotin	Brewer's yeast, brown rice, cashew nuts, cheese, chicken, eggs, lentils, mackerel, meat, milk, oats, peanuts, peas, soya beans, sunflower seeds, tuna, walnuts
Calcium	Almonds, Brazil nuts, cheese, kelp, milk, molasses, salmon (canned), sardines (canned), shrimp, soya beans, yogurt
Carbohydrates	Bread, corn, crackers, noodles, oats, pasta, potatoes, rice, sweet potatoes
Chromium	Beef, brewer's yeast, chicken, eggs, fish, fruit, milk products, potatoes, whole grains
Coenzyme Q10	All foods, particularly, beef, mackerel, sardines, soya oil, spinach
Essential fatty acids (EFAs)	Oily fish (e.g. mackerel, salmon, sardines, tuna); flax, sesame, pumpkin and sunflower seeds and their unprocessed oils
Fibre	Barley, beans (e.g. borlotti, pinto, kidney, black-eyed, chickpeas), brown rice, buckwheat, fresh fruit, fresh vegetables, lentils, oats, rye, wholewheat

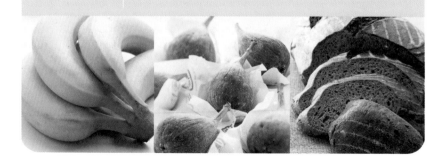

NUTRIENTS AND THEIR RICH FOOD SOURCES

NUTRIENT	RICH FOOD SOURCES
Folic acid	Barley, brewer's yeast, fruits, chickpeas, green leafy vegetables, lentils, peas, rice, soya beans, whole wheat, wheatgerm
Iodine	Cod-liver oil, fish, oysters, table salt (iodized), seaweed, sunflower seeds
Iron	Cashew nuts, cheese, egg yolk, chickpeas, lentils, molasses, mussels, pumpkin seeds, seaweed, walnuts, wheatgerm, whole grains
Magnesium	Almonds, fish, green leafy vegetables, kelp, molasses, nuts, soya beans, sunflower seeds, wheatgerm
Manganese	Avocados, barley, blackberries, buckwheat, chestnuts, ginger, hazelnuts, oats, peas, pecans, seaweed, spinach
Potassium	Avocados, bananas, citrus fruits, lentils, milk, molasses, nuts, parsnips, potatoes, raisins, sardines (canned), spinach, whole grains
Protein	Dairy products, eggs, fish, meat, poultry, soya
Selenium	Broccoli, cabbage, celery, chicken, egg yolk, garlic, liver, milk, mushrooms, onions, seafood, wheatgerm, whole grains
Sodium	Bacon, bread, butter, canned vegetables, ham, milk, table salt and most commercially processed and packaged foods
Sulphur	Cabbage, clams, eggs, fish, garlic, milk, onions, wheatgerm
Zinc	Egg yolk, fish, all meat, milk, molasses, oysters, sesame seeds, soya beans, sunflower seeds, turkey, wheatgerm, whole grains

FEEL-GOOD STRATEGIES

Although this book focuses primarily on the nutritional aspects of improving mood, many other forms of therapy can make a significant difference to how you feel. Looking after your body and mind should be a holistic experience that encompasses all aspects of what it is to be alive.

A healthy, balanced diet is a great starting point from which to address any mood-related problems you may be experiencing. However, your strategies for feeling better should not be limited to dietary changes. There are a host of additional ways of boosting your moods that involve looking beyond your body's nutritional needs. For example, appropriate, regular exercise can have a profound, long-lasting positive effect on your physical and emotional well-being.

Similarly, sharing problems with a family member, friend or professional therapist often leaves you feeling lighter and more at ease with yourself. You may choose to try one of the wide range of complementary therapies that can ease physical and mental symptoms, and also help you to relax and rediscover harmony between your body and mind. The alternative therapies covered here include acupuncture, homoeopathy, herbal medicine, flower essences, aromatherapy and massage.

GET MOVING

Consider that one way of looking at low moods and fatigue is as negative energy in your body and mind, dragging you down. If you exercise, you are taking that negative energy and transforming it into a positive, life-enhancing force. However you choose to look at it, there is no getting away from the fact that exercise does make you feel better (*see* box, opposite). Any lifestyle aimed at getting or maintaining a healthy body and mind must involve some sort of regular physical activity. It is something all of us are aware of, some of us do without fail, some of us get round to intermittently (and then remember how great it feels) and some of us ignore completely. Unless you are in the first category and therefore need no encouragement at all, the key to incorporating regular exercise into your weekly routine is to choose a form of physical activity that stimulates you, one you enjoy and one that is appropriate for your level of strength and fitness.

Exercise may consist of very simple activities, even just stretching at home. If you are unfit, suddenly going to the gym and spending 45 minutes on the treadmill, even if you could manage it, would not be the best thing for you. In fact, your body would

THE BENEFITS OF EXERCISE

Taking appropriate exercise in combination with a balanced diet is one of the most powerful forms of natural medicine for a healthy mind and body. The effects are cumulative. Here are just some of the benefits of regular exercise:

- balances blood sugar and helps reduce cravings
- improves cholesterol, lowers blood pressure and inflammatory markers
- improves metabolism by boosting the number and function of mitochondria (components within cells that help with the production of energy)
- improves mood and concentration
- improves sleep and relieves stress and anxiety
- balances sex hormones and improves production of human growth hormone and DHEA known to have anti-ageing benefits
- improves body image and shape, increasing muscle mass and decreasing fat

probably feel quite distressed. It is therefore very important to choose a form of exercise that is appropriate for you – it should be something that you will enjoy, the prospect of which is going to encourage you (at least most of the time), and which is not going to feel like a chore.

Pushing yourself too hard is not helpful and may ultimately make you feel worse (studies have shown that even in very fit athletes, over-training can bring on depression and exhaustion). Start with a gentle activity, such as swimming or jogging, or perhaps take up a one-on-one game, such as badminton or tennis. Consider joining a team (as long as the level is appropriate to you) – playing a team sport, even once a week, can really make you feel like part of a network. On the other hand, you may be happiest going for a brisk walk by yourself or with your dog. Listening to music while you exercise – be it energizing or relaxing – can also contribute to the benefits if it means that you enjoy the experience more. Basically, go for whatever suits you.

Unfortunately, when you are feeling low emotionally you often lack the motivation to exercise (let's face it, even many people who are not depressed find it difficult to bring themselves to partake in some physical activity). In such a case, you may find it helpful to arrange to exercise with a friend, so that you can encourage one another.

Once you have started to exercise, the benefits you will feel are likely to act as an incentive for you to make it a regular event. Don't give up if it is tough at first – often you have to almost force yourself to get started, in order to break the cycle of lethargy, but only then will the feeling of improved mood and higher energy come.

TIPS FOR GETTING MOVING

The first step in beginning an exercise programme is the all-important decision to get moving. Once you are feeling motivated you will be keen to discover and enjoy the benefits that exercise can bring. Bear these tips in mind, make sure you are well prepared, and go for it!

* Check with your doctor first if you have any doubt about your ability to exercise, for example if you have reason to be worried about your cardiac health, or suffer from any bone or muscle problems.
* Always start gently and build up slowly. If you are exercising at a club or in a class, talk to your trainer or teacher about what is best for you.
* For fat loss it is best to exercise on an empty stomach – ideally first thing in the morning. Eat a protein-based breakfast within 45 minutes of finishing your exercise to help refuel your muscles and balance blood sugar. However, there's no point in dragging yourself out of bed 90 minutes earlier than usual if it is just going to make you feel more exhausted and miserable. You should exercise at the time of day that feels right for you – just be careful not to exercise late at night as this can interfere with sleep patterns.
* Try to exercise outdoors in daylight as this will naturally increase your levels of vitamin D, which can help boost your mood.
* Keeping yourself flexible and supple will help prevent injury, muscle soreness and stiffness. Aim to include stretching after an exercise session or take up yoga or Pilates.
* Even if it is hard to get yourself going, it is important that you actually want to exercise, so choose an activity that inspires you and surround it with motivating add-ons, such as music and wearing comfortable, appropriate clothing/shoes.
* Exercising with a friend can help to motivate you.
* Exercise need not be fancy and expensive and require special gear. Even walking can be an excellent form of exercise: you can do it anywhere and it's free. Walking for just 20 minutes a day can make a difference. You could even incorporate it in your journey to work, your lunch break or going to pick up the children from school. Make sure you walk in a safe area that is well lit if you walk at night.

There are several forms of exercise which, although not directly considered aerobic, provide a remarkably good workout for the body at the same time as relaxing your mind. Most of these forms of exercise come from Eastern traditions – they include yoga or any of the martial arts-based forms, such as tai chi and qigong. At the same time as invigorating your body, they can calm your mind in an extremely powerful and meditative way.

TALK IT THROUGH

The old saying "a problem shared is a problem halved", like many such adages, has more than a grain of truth in it. If there is something playing on your mind, getting it out of your own head can often do wonders to dissipate the negativity it can create.

Sometimes it can really help to turn to a partner, friend or colleague to externalize a persistent thought, worry or concern – in doing so, you often obtain a broader perspective or an alternative viewpoint that helps to make the problem easier to cope with. At other times, you may feel that it would be easier to talk your worries through with a virtual stranger, someone more removed from your life, in which case seeking support from a professional therapist (*see* below) or life coach (*see* box, page 189) may be more useful. Either way, taking the step of admitting that you need support is often the highest hurdle to overcome. It can be very empowering to realize that reaching out for help is not only a sign of strength, but also a very normal, healthy human reaction.

BRIDGING THE GAP

Because low moods are very often precipitated by low self-esteem, a traumatic event, chronic stress in domestic or working life, repeated destructive behavioural patterns or internalized anger, it is usually very helpful to break such patterns, to learn to deal with certain situations or to learn to accept oneself. After all, life is always going to present us with difficulties, and it is how we perceive these and how we handle them that makes the difference. Talking therapies, such as counselling or some sort of psychotherapy, can be extremely useful in such situations. If you embark on such a programme, bear in mind that therapy does not offer a "cure", is not always easy and often involves a long-term investment of time and effort. However, your therapist can lend a non-judgmental, listening ear along the journey and the rewards, in terms of your emotional well-being, can be considerable.

Many scientific trials have tested the efficacy of talking therapies compared with antidepressant medication. Several studies have shown cognitive therapy, for example, to be more effective than medication, while others have suggested that cognitive therapy adds to the efficacy of drug treatment. (Cognitive therapy addresses the cognitions – perception, intuition, reactions – that mediate the impact of events in a person's life.)

Exploring acceptance, self-worth and how one deals with life events can be invaluable in overcoming persistent or recurring low moods or depression. Even if all biochemical imbalances are corrected, the mind's delicate equilibrium can be easily upset by negative behavioural patterns and reaction to stressors.

There are countless types of psychotherapy to choose from, but it appears that it is not the particular school of training that makes the most difference, but the strength of the bond between the therapist and client.

OTHER APPROACHES

For many of us with busy lifestyles, making time for ourselves is surprisingly difficult, and it is often something we relegate to the bottom of our list of priorities. However, "me time" is crucial to balancing everything else that is going on in our lives.

When you are feeling down, there are countless simple ways to give yourself a boost. Just taking some time out from your daily routine to relax and rejuvenate your body and mind – whether that be in the form of having a bath, playing with the children or doing some exercise – can make a tremendous difference.

If you have been feeling persistently low for a long time, in addition to adopting the nutritional strategies described in this book, you may also want to try a complementary therapy that addresses stress-related problems and helps you to rediscover harmony between your body and mind. With the recent emergence of more and more variations of all sorts of therapies, there are plenty to choose from, including the ones discussed below.

ACUPUNCTURE

This is the ancient Eastern art of using very fine needles, which are painlessly inserted into special points along meridians (energy lines) in the body, gently to correct imbalances in the body's natural energy flow. A very powerful treatment, acupuncture can help deal with both physical and mental conditions. Some scientific trials have found acupuncture to be at least as effective as drug therapy in combating depression.

HOMOEOPATHY

This is one of the truly holistic therapies that, although seemingly incredibly subtle, can have remarkable effects. You are given a specifically chosen remedy by your homoeopath – in an infinitesimal dosage – which stimulates the body to heal imbalances.

HERBAL MEDICINE

Both the traditional Chinese and Western use of plants for medical purposes are almost as old as humankind itself. In the West, the best-known herb for helping balance mood is St John's wort, which is among the most widely prescribed antidepressants in Germany. It is believed to work by increasing the levels of serotonin in circu-

LIFE COACHING

If the thought of entering into a therapy programme of any sort does not appeal, perhaps life coaching would be more appropriate for you. Working with a life coach can give you the confidence and ability to move forward in the areas of your life where you feel you are in a rut. Life coaches recognize that it is often our own frustrations and sense of stagnation, along with our failure to realize our own potential, that can leave us feeling low. A professional life coach, who can often provide sessions by telephone or email, can help you in several ways. He or she may:

- show you how to set more appropriate, realistic goals and then reach them
- encourage you to achieve more by working on ways to take down the barriers to doing so
- help you to focus better, to produce results more efficiently
- provide you with the tools, support and structure to improve any area of your life

lation in the body. It is best to visit a qualified medical herbalist who can give you a prescription for this, or other herbs tailored to your personal needs.

FLOWER ESSENCES

Flower essences are another very subtle but effective way of correcting a wide range of emotional imbalances. You can buy flower essences at most health shops and chemists, and there are several books available that can help you choose which essences would be most appropriate for you. However, as with herbal and aromatherapy remedies, flower essences are best taken under the guidance of an experienced health practitioner.

AROMATHERAPY

The concentrated essential oils of plants are used for massage, inhalation, compresses, baths and in special burners. When chosen by a trained aromatherapist, the blend of oils used can help to relieve a range of both emotional and physical conditions.

MASSAGE

There are many types of massage available – from aromatherapy, to deep tissue to shiatsu. The best way to find out which is suited to you is to contact a local natural health clinic and discuss your wants and needs. When performed by a skilled practitioner, massage can have very profound physical and emotional effects.

GLOSSARY

ACETYLCHOLINE

The main **neurotransmitter** for communication between brain **neurons** that is responsible for, among other things, memory and cognitive thinking.

ADRENALIN

Also known as epinephrine, this hormone is secreted by the adrenal glands as part of the body's response to stress. Adrenalin plays a role in effecting physiological changes that include faster breathing, raised heart rate and increased levels of blood **glucose**, all of which are intended to enable the body to respond effectively to a stressful situation.

AMINO ACID

A building block of **protein**. All the proteins in the body are made up of combinations of any number of amino acids, of which there are about twenty in total.

ANTIOXIDANT

A substance – nutrient or enzyme – which can "disarm" an **oxidant**. In other words, antioxidants neutralize the potentially damaging effects of oxidation. Key antioxidant **nutrients** are vitamins A, C and E. Fresh fruit and vegetables, nuts, seeds and whole grains are all particularly rich sources of antioxidants.

CARBOHYDRATE

A sugar or starch which is used by the body primarily as fuel for energy production. Rice, pasta, bread, potatoes and sugar are rich sources of carbohydrates.

CORTISOL

A hormone secreted by the adrenal glands in response to stress. Cortisol plays a part in effecting the physiological changes that help the body deal with the stress, perceived or real. One of cortisol's key roles is to increase the supply of **glucose** to the brain and other tissues. Cortisol helps reduce inflammation, but also appears to interfere with the levels of the mood-boosting **neurotransmitters serotonin** and **dopamine** that the body produces naturally.

DHA

DHA, or docosahexaenoic acid, is an **essential fatty acid** found in fish, and can also be produced in the body from fats contained in flaxseeds (linseeds), hemp seeds and walnuts. DHA is used in the body in the lining of nerves and cell membranes.

DOPAMINE

Like **serotonin**, dopamine is a **neurotransmitter** involved in mood and motivation. Dopamine can be made in the body from the amino acids phenylalanine and tyrosine.

EPA

EPA, or eicosapentaenoic acid, is an **essential fatty acid** that is in the same "family" as **DHA**. EPA is found in fish, and can also be made in the body from fats contained in flaxseeds (linseeds), hemp seeds and walnuts. EPA has many uses in the body, including forming part of the lining of nerves and cell membranes.

ESSENTIAL FATTY ACIDS (EFAs)

A group of fats (oils) essential for many vital functions in the body, including healthy brain and nerve cells, balanced hormones, energy production and well-hydrated skin. EFAs can only be obtained from your diet; rich sources are nuts, seeds and oily fish.

GLUCOSE

A type of sugar that is the prime source of fuel for energy in the brain as well as the rest of the body. The body converts **carbohydrates** into sugars such as glucose during the digestive process.

GLUTEN

A **protein** found in grains such as wheat, oats, rye and barley.

GLYCAEMIC INDEX

A scale that measures the rate at which a particular food is digested and released as **glucose** into the bloodstream. The faster a food raises blood-sugar levels, the higher it is rated on the GI scale.

GLYCAEMIC LOAD

Related to **glycaemic index**, the glycaemic load of a food takes account both of its GI and the amount eaten. A food's GL is calculated by multiplying its GI score by the amount of carbohydrate per serving.

NEURON

A nerve cell, sometimes called a neurone. Nerve cells exist throughout the body and brain.

NEUROTRANSMITTER

A chemical in the body that facilitates the transmission of impulses (messages) through the nervous system, from one **neuron** to the next.

NUTRIENTS

All chemical reactions that take place in the body depend on a regular supply of "micro" nutrients, such as vitamins and minerals, and "macro" nutrients, including **protein, carbohydrates**, fats and water.

OXIDANTS

Molecules that are by-products of oxygen and can be likened to "sparks" from anything that burns, including cigarettes and food, as well as the combustion of **glucose** in our cells to make energy. Oxidants can damage cells, thereby accelerating ageing and causing disease. **Antioxidants** help counter such damage.

PHOSPHATIDYL CHOLINE (PC)

A type of **phospholipid** containing choline, which is incorporated into healthy cell membranes and is needed to make **acetylcholine**. PC is also contained in bile where it contributes to the proper digestion of fats. Lecithin (found in soya, eggs and as a food supplement) is a source of PC.

PHOSPHATIDYL SERINE (PS)

A type of **phospholipid** that is an essential component of human cell membranes. PS, which is thought to play an important role in the body's **neurotransmitter** function, is found in small amounts in soya lecithin and is also available as a food supplement.

PHOSPHOLIPID

A substance made of phosphorus
and lipids (fats), phospholipid forms
an important part of human cell
membranes, including those of **neurons**.

PROBIOTICS

A term used to describe the so-called
"bacteria", such as Lactobacillus
acidophilus and bifidobacteria, that are
needed for healthy digestion. Probiotics
are available as food supplements and
are also found in live, natural yogurt.

PROTEIN

Made of **amino acids**, proteins are used
in the body to form the main structures,
including all cells, as well as enzymes,
hormones and **neurotransmitters**. Fish,
poultry, meat, milk, yogurt, cheese and
beans are rich sources of protein.

SATURATED FAT

A type of fat found mainly in animal-
derived foods such as meat and dairy
products.

SEROTONIN

A mood-boosting **neurotransmitter** that
is involved in numerous processes in the
body, including sending out the signals
that control appetite. Serotonin is derived
from the **amino acid tryptophan**.

TRANS FAT

A type of fat that has been transformed
by exposure to excess heat or light,
changing its chemical structure and
rendering it harmful to the body. **EFAs**
are susceptible to oxidation damage,
which can turn them into trans fats.

Many commercially produced oils and
processed foods contain trans fats.

TRYPTOPHAN

An **amino acid** that is particularly
abundant in bananas, chicken, figs, milk,
seaweeds, sunflower seeds, tuna, turkey
and yogurt. Tryptophan can be converted
in the body into the **neurotransmitter
serotonin**.

UNSATURATED FAT

Unsaturated fats are found in vegetable
sources, including oils such as olive,
sunflower, safflower, rapeseed, soya,
peanut and sesame. Unsaturated
fats can be further subdivided into
monounsaturated and polyunsaturated
fats (the latter is another name for
essential fatty acids).

RESOURCES

IN THE UK:

British Association for Applied Nutrition and Nutritional Therapy (BANT)
27 Old Gloucester Street
London WC1N 3XX
Tel: 0870 606 1284
www.bant.org.uk

British Association for Counselling and Psychotherapy (BACP)
BACP House
15 St John's Business Park
Lutterworth, Leicestershire LE17 4HB
Tel: 01455 883300
www.bacp.co.uk

UK Council for Psychotherapy (UKCP)
2nd Floor, Edward House
2 Wakley Street, London EC1V 7LT
Tel: 020 7014 9955
www.psychotherapy.org.uk

The London Sleep Centre
137 Harley Street, London W1G 6BF
Tel: 020 7725 2523
www.londonsleepcentre.com

British Allergy Foundation
Allergy UK, LEFA Business Park
Edgington Way, Sidcup, Kent DA14 5BH
Tel: 01322 619898
www.allergyuk.org

IN AUSTRALIA & NEW ZEALAND:

Australasian College of Nutritional & Environmental Medicine Inc (ACNEM)
Suite 10, 23–25 Melrose Street
Sandringham, Victoria, 3191
Tel: (0)3 9597 0363
www.acnem.org

Australian Natural Therapists' Association (ANTA)
PO Box 657, Maroochydore
Queensland 4558
Tel: 1800 817 577
www.australiannaturaltherapists
association.com.au

South Pacific Association of Natural Therapists (SPANT)
28 Willow Avenue, Birkenhead
Auckland 1310
Tel: (0)9 445 7885

FURTHER READING

Bailey, Christine *The Juice Diet* (Duncan Baird Publishers), 2011
Bailey, Christine *The Raw Food Diet* (Duncan Baird Publishers), 2012
Bailey, Christine *The Top 100 Recipes for Brainy Kids* (Duncan Baird Publishers), 2009
Crawford Michael et. al. *Nutrition and Mental Health: A Handbook* (Pavillion), 2008
Glenville, Marilyn *The Natural Health Bible for Women* (Duncan Baird Publishers), 2010
Glenville, Marilyn *Natural Solutions to Menopause* (Rodale), 2011
Holford, Patrick *The Feel Good Factor* (Piatkus), 2010
Hyman, Mark *The Blood Sugar Solution* (Hodder & Stoughton), 2012
Savona, Natalie *The Big Book of Juices and Smoothies* (Duncan Baird Publishers), 2003
Watts, Martina (ed.) *Nutrition and Addiction* (Pavillion), 2011

INDEX

Entries in *italics* indicate recipes